KETO

FOR WOMEN OVER 50:

A Complete Guide to Keto Diet for Women Over 50. Understanding Nutritional Needs for Weight Management and Health Improvement.

CAREN HEAL

Table of Contents

Introduction

As a woman enters her fifties, it becomes necessary to make modifications to the diet to be healthy. This is because of changes in hormones and metabolism. There is a decrease in muscle mass. To offset this change, there is a need to increase the amount of protein in the diet. At the same time, bone density decreases, making it necessary to increase the amount of vitamin D and calcium consumed in order to maintain adequate bone density as the body ages. All this, combined with a reduction in the number of calories needed to fuel the body, makes it necessary to modify diet as a woman enters postmenopausal years. These natural changes to the body make changes to the diet necessary as a woman ages.

Because of the changes occurring in the bodies of women over 50, it is imperative to look at how the needs of these women are different than younger women and men. During menopause, hormones shift in women, and these changes make it necessary to make some adjustments to their lifestyle in general, and diet in particular.

Also, as women age, their ability to discern thirstiness may diminish. Water consumption is still an important factor in the health of a woman. Because it is harder to determine thirst as you surpass your 50th year, it is essential that you consume 8 to 9 8 oz glasses of water each day. Drink more in the winter in hot weather and when exercising. While you are drinking more water, it may serve to curb your appetite. This is good because you will need to lower your caloric intake from what you may be accustomed to. This happens when you are finding new aches and pains and slowing down your exercise regime. Exercise may be less intense as you make modifications to coincide with your age and decreases in mobility. This is because you are not as flexible and may be experiencing inflammation in your joints. While these are all relatively normal signs of aging, the decrease in physical activity may cause additional problems in the form of weight gain.

This may be a good time to eliminate processed foods and sugar from your diet. Dietary fiber is the key to avoiding constipation. Studies show that women over 50 may be up to seven times more likely to suffer from constipation than men of a similar age. Failure to consume enough dietary fiber can result in a small, hard stool. It is beneficial to consume dietary fiber, which is found in whole grains, and food is made from whole grains, as well as fruits and vegetables. The foods move through intestines easily and make a solid stool that moves through the intestines quickly and efficiently. The dietary fiber in these foods may help in lowering bad cholesterol (LDL) levels in adults. This may have a positive effect on heart health as well. Since estrogen levels in women are also decreasing, the female body begins to lose the positive effect estrogen has on the heart and blood vessels. This is another impact of menopause. Consuming adequate amounts of dietary fiber may help to improve heart health.

Women over 50 may want to modify their keto approach by increasing the daily carbohydrates to 100 to 150 g each day. They may also want to increase the protein from 25% to 30% of the diet. The remaining amount of food will be fat. The increased carbohydrates provide less distress to hormones and metabolism and put less stress on the body while adjusting to a diet low in carbohydrates. The increase in protein is to offset the body's tendency to lose muscle mass as women age. Additionally, the carbs will provide energy to exercise. The metabolism of women typically slow as women age. The increase in carbs and protein may allow women over 50 to forgo the sluggish feelings and allow enough energy to exercise while on the diet. This will improve overall health.

Carbohydrates in your diet should come from whole grains or high-quality carbs like pumpkins, carrots, spaghetti squash, and small quantities of butternut squash. Foods that grow below the ground have higher carbohydrate content. If you feel like you need to sneak them into your diet, it should be small amounts per serving. They add variety and flavor to your diet, but they must be used in moderation. Even with a few extra carbs in your diet, you should be able to enter ketosis. The same is true for protein. The body may not enter ketosis as quickly, but the effects of the changes will not be as jarring to your body and the internal system of operation.

CHAPTER 1:

How To Start When You Are Over 50

Like any other life-transforming endeavor, the keto diet regimen is dependent on your mindset. You must be prepared to face the emotional, physical, and psychological obstacles that will arise in the course of achieving your goals. This underpins the impact the diet will have on your life. In this regard, one of the fundamental elements of keto is a mindset that is equipped to deal with many obstacles and challenges.

At this point, you will encounter an in-depth analysis and discussion of the right keto-diet mindset as well as how to achieve it. While the keto diet proves challenging for any person, an even greater challenge emerges for women above 50. The decision to transform your diet often arises from a myriad of reasons.

For some, the desire to lose weight is the underlying impetus, while others are motivated by the goal of living healthier lives. In some cases, a person may be forced to consider a diet change for medical or biological reasons. Regardless of the motivation, maintaining the right mindset always determines the success of a change in diet. In this regard, attaining an appropriate mindset is the first step towards initiating and benefitting from a keto-based diet.

Having read and heard about the keto diet for ages, you may now find it necessary to do keto in your life. With pictures and images available on the Internet regarding its amazing outcomes, one is often pumped up and ready to start it in their life. However, it is important to move beyond the hype you see on social media channels surrounding the keto diet.

The Right Mindset

When beginning a keto diet, the first phase of your journey must be adopting an appropriate mindset that will allow you to make this lifestyle change successfully. While you might set your goals right from the start, you must consider that your energy and enthusiasm is likely to wane over time. For most people, this results in failure, which is then translated into frustration and the loss of confidence in the ketogenic diet. By emotionally and psychologically preparing oneself for the journey ahead, it is possible to achieve this feat quite easily.

You must first acknowledge and accept in your mind that the diet does work and that you can experience its impact on your life. This is the first and most crucial thought process that will help you actively and judiciously stick to the plan. If you have tried other diet plans in the past with little success, this particular thought process may be hard to come by. However, by shifting your focus to scientific and factual material regarding the diet, you may begin to appreciate its efficacy.

The capacity to individually internalize this concept forms the basis of the essential mindset for a keto diet. By eliminating any form of doubt in your mind with respect to the benefits and impact of a keto diet, you set yourself up for success. This is because it helps you stay focused on the outcome while ignoring the day to day challenges and distractions that will surely arise. Internalization and appreciation of the benefits and effectiveness of the keto diet create the necessary momentum needed to consistently adhere to the stipulations that come with the implementation of the diet.

The elimination of excuses is also fundamental if you are to realize the benefits of a keto diet. For most people, dietary changes are seen as major transformations that occur overnight. For a woman in her 50s, this can prove daunting and even scary. When you have already lived on a different diet for half a century, you have an internal block that causes you to doubt your ability to change the content of your diet. You are likely to come up with numerous excuses and justifications as to why such a diet may not work for you. If you are looking at a keto diet as a total overhaul of how you are a person, then there is a higher likelihood you will find the endeavor too arduous to even try.

By holding onto the notion a keto diet is only successful when drastic and dramatic changes are made in your life, you hold yourself back with your own thoughts. In most cases, this line of thought should raise the red flag of fear and unnecessary excuses. While such notions may have been informed by your preceding attempts at dieting, it is important that you approach a keto diet with a fresh and inquisitive mind.

Diet and lifestyle transformations are not achieved overnight, and neither do they require tremendous resources for their actualization. To set yourself up for success, you must be ready to begin where you are and with what you have. The willingness to start is what matters the most. This will make it possible for eventual success even as you gradually work towards your goal.

As you gradually advance to your goal of diet change, you are likely to enjoy the small victories, and you will notice that over time, you will be able to draw inspiration from the hurdles and obstacles that arise along the way.

It is also important to approach the keto diet as a new partner that will bring you much-awaited love, compassion, and care. In other words, you have to understand and appreciate the fact the keto diet is there to transform your life like never before. In this case, therefore, you must assume a sense of self-love and care to ensure that it works. Day-to-day interactions and experiences can often impose a sense of negativity and self-loathing. In failing to accomplish various goals, meet specific demands, or accomplish certain personal, professional, or social goals, the burden of guilt and self-hate is likely to emerge.

Such a state of mind is limited in numerous ways, and as such, it cannot achieve the desired frequency of caring for itself. Once you learn to be kind and patient with yourself, you realize life has its ups and downs. Regardless of these challenges, you must give yourself the time and space to fail, learn, and grow as you go. The self-care mindset is crucial for effectiveness on the keto diet. By appreciating and loving yourself, you initiate a process in which your well-being is paramount to your survival, and as such, you are ready to undertake any efforts whatsoever to improve the quality of your life. A sense of purpose and limitlessness becomes a constant aspect of your life, and as such, you are able to see your goals and ambitions through.

As is the case, with most new things, encounters, and experiences, you are likely to feel the need to continuously remind yourself of the feeling. For instance, when you buy a new phone, you may not want to put it down even as you explore its features and quirks. Over time your adoration for the new item may turn into an obsession or compulsive behavior that can be hard to break. The same analogy works when it comes to dieting. In setting out to try a new diet, as is the case with a keto diet, you may fixate on the expected outcomes and results.

In other words, your primary goal may involve constantly checking your weight to check the progress being made. Tracking your weight all the time sets you up for failure, considering the dynamics of a keto diet. As you initiate a ketogenic diet, you must remember that the impact of years of an unchecked diet cannot be eliminated within weeks or sometimes even months.

In other words, weight loss and improved health may not be evident within the first few weeks or even months for some people. While you may watch how you eat, change your lifestyle, and even adopt a training regime, the results will be slow and gradual. By fixating on lost pounds, therefore, you are likely to get disappointed and end up abandoning the entire process.

It is important to note the fact that while your weight may be slow to change, there is a likelihood your muscle structure will have a change in terms of getting leaner. By moving away from the metric-tracking mentality, you allow yourself the time to acclimate to the diet and notice the overall changes it brings about in your physical, psychological, and emotional well-being rather than fixating on the pounds lost or gained.

Cognitively preparing for the long-haul is also vital in achieving the goals and benefits of a keto diet.

The best way to appreciate a ketogenic diet is by looking at it as a lifestyle change rather than a change in dietary intakes. While the benefits of the diet are factual and well documented, they take time to come about. Most people, however, hold the belief that a keto diet is a quick fix solution that allows them to transform their health, weight, and body shape within weeks or months. Having gleaned information from various media platforms, such individuals are quick to adopt the diet with the hope of having an overnight transformation.

The quick-fix mindset is one of the surest ways of failing in your pursuit to experience the benefits of a ketogenic diet. You must be willing to endure for the long-term goals while celebrating the short-term gains. A two-week on a two-month keto diet may accord you the much need weight loss. However, such changes are likely to disappear just as fast in the absence of long-term commitment.

CHAPTER 2:

Organization Of The Day

Step 1

Calculate and track your macros. Macronutrients (macros) are carbohydrates, fats, and proteins. An average person would need more fat and fewer carbs, while a professional athlete may need more protein and high carbohydrate consumption.

Track your calorie consumption. Skipping a meal here or there is not harmful when it is occasional but restricting calories for longer periods can have negative effects on your health. Carb cycling also involves calorie cycling so you can switch from low-calorie to higher-calorie periods.

Keep an eye on the amount of cholesterol. If your cholesterol level is high, avoid saturated fats (found primarily in red meat) and opt for monounsaturated fats. Trans fats such as partially hydrogenated vegetable oils are out of the question; they can be found in margarine and other spreads, fried foods, packaged foods, and fast foods. On the other hand, you should increase soluble fiber, foods rich in omega-3 fatty acid (herring, salmon, mackerel, flaxseeds, and walnuts).

Replenish electrolytes. Just make sure that you are eating foods that contain electrolytes such as bouillon, leafy green, avocado, and Himalayan salt. Taking magnesium supplements may be beneficial on a keto diet.

A few more tips. Consume at least eight glasses of water per day to stay hydrated on the ketogenic diet. Further, get regular exercise. It does not have to be anything special and time-consuming. Simply find an activity that fits into your schedule like walking, cycling, or stair climbing. Keep it simple since the ketogenic diet requires a little pre-planning. Stick to real and nutrient-dense foods and find good alternatives for your favorite carbs. I am sure you will find inspiration and motivation in these six hundred recipes. You will learn how to prepare keto pancakes, granola, desserts, waffles, and snacks. It is all about variety and smart food choices, not rigid rules, and restrictive diet plans. And remember – you are beautiful just the way you are, take a deep breath and love yourself.

Weigh Your Food: Being accurate about your macros is very crucial to the success of the ketogenic diet. Make sure that you invest in a good food scale so that you can monitor your macro intake. So, avoid the guesswork and use a scale to measure your food. If you have more money to spare, buy scales that you can connect to apps and websites.

• Drink Water: Staying hydrated is one of the most important rules when it comes to following any kind of diet regimen. Start your day by consuming at least 8 to 16 ounces of water to allow the body to begin its natural cycle.

• Exercise: Remember that diet alone will not help you lose as much weight as you want. You can also do resistant training because it requires more protein to aid in muscle gain. This exercise is great for keeping your protein in check especially if you consumed more of it than fats. Make sure that you match this diet regimen with a high interval and high-intensity workout to improve your blood glucose levels. Exercise at least 25 minutes every day to see the best results.

• Reduce Your Stress: Stress can affect your hormone levels by causing your blood sugar level to rise thus increasing your cravings. Have you ever noticed why you often crave sweets when you are stressed out? That is your hormone talking. While you cannot control the stress that comes your way, find ways on how to mitigate it. You can practice yoga, mindfulness, and breathing exercises to take away your stress.

• Choose Quality Carbs: Some of you may say that carb is carb no matter what form they exist in. But remember that not all carbs are created equally. There are carbs that are nutrient-rich and are found in non-starchy vegetables and some fruits. So, when making a meal plan, make sure that you use good quality carbs.

• Stay Away from Diet Soda: Just because it comes with the word "diet" with it does not mean that it is good for you. Diet soda uses a wide variety of sugar substitutes that tells your body that is has an overload of sugar thereby shutting the metabolism down. So, if you need to quench your thirst, drink sparkling water instead.

• Get Enough Sleep: Sleep is necessary for you to lose weight fast. Remember that the lack of sleep causes stress to the body. Stress can affect the hormone levels in your body thus increasing your cravings to constantly snack on food. So, make sure that you get at least 6 to 8 hours of sleep daily.

• Intermittent Fasting: If you genuinely want to lose weight fast with the ketogenic diet, you might want to consider pairing it with intermittent fasting. Intermittent fasting is when you fast for more than 12 hours so that your body will use up the stored fats as its primary fuel. Consume your keto-friendly meals within a short eating window time and the rest of the day should be dedicated to no food consumption so that your body can undergo the state of ketosis faster. For instance, you can go fasting from 2:00 pm to 8:00 am the following day. From 8:01 am to 1:59 pm, that is the only time you allow yourself to eat your meals.

Step 2

You must remember that just like all other diet regimens, not everyone can follow a ketogenic diet. So, before you start this regimen, ask yourself if the ketogenic diet is really for you? Below are the things that you should consider seeing if the ketogenic diet is for you.

• How long can I follow this diet? The ketogenic diet is not like your usual fad diet only lasting for a few weeks. To see results, it will take you months or even a year. So, if you are someone who cannot follow its principles long-term, then this diet is not for you.

• Will the eating plan fit my food preference, budget needs, and culture? If you follow a strict dietary guideline (veganism or vegetarianism) then you might need to tweak the ketogenic diet to fit your preferences. It may difficult, but not impossible. However, if you find it too much of a hassle to tweak the ketogenic meal plan to fit your preference, you might not enjoy this diet at all.

• Do I have medical conditions that will put me at risk? While the ketogenic diet has therapeutic effects on people who suffer from diabetes and cardiovascular diseases, it is not prescribed among people who suffer from kidney-related problems as the presence of protein and fats can be damaging to the kidneys.

The bottom line is that while the ketogenic diet is good for most people, it may not be advisable for some. So, before you ask yourself if this diet is for you, make sure that you seek advice from your nutritionist or physician.

Since the carbohydrate intake for this diet is kept at an exceptionally low, carbs are practically absent thus the body is pushed to utilize other forms of energy in the form of fat.

 In the absence of fat, the liver takes the fatty acids in the body then converts it into ketone bodies. You must remember that the body just cannot take fat and use it in its raw form. It must undergo different processes so that it can be utilized effectively by the body. This is the reason why it needs to convert it into ketone form. This process is called ketosis, and this is what the ketogenic diet is all about.

 In a nutshell, there are three types of ketone bodies created during the break down of fatty acids and these include (1) acetoacetate, (2) beta-hydroxybutyric acid, and (3) acetone.

There are numerous benefits of the keto diet aside from weight loss and better energy levels.

• Better blood sugar control: The ketogenic diet lowers the blood sugar levels thus making it a great way to manage or even prevent diabetes. The thing is that the body takes a rest from producing insulin t;hus it can stabilize itself during ketosis.

- Improved mental focus: Several studies suggest that the ketogenic diet can increase health performance. Because this diet does not spike blood sugar levels, the brain is kept in a stable condition. Moreover, the brain simply loves ketones as its primary source of fuel.

- Reduced cravings and hunger pains: Fats are known to be filling, so this diet does not only curb your cravings but also reduces hunger pains.

- Better cholesterol and blood pressure levels: This diet regimen can improve triglyceride and cholesterol levels in the body. This reduces the risk of developing clogged arteries.

- Clearer skin: Didn't you know that the ketogenic diet can help improve the quality of your skin? Several studies suggest that people who follow the ketogenic diet often experience clearing of their acne and other skin anomalies. The ketogenic diet, aside from pushing ketosis, also drives the immune system into a frenzy thus it can help eliminate inflammation on the skin.

Before you can experience the many benefits of the ketogenic diet, it is important that you eat mostly fat. But how much fat is too much? When I first started, I had this misinformed idea that all I need to do is to eat all the fatty foods that I see. This was easy as pie, I said. And to tell you the truth, I see countless dieters out there who make the same mistake that I did.

To succeed with the ketogenic diet, you do not need to eat a lot of fat. Rather, you need to smartly break down what you eat to 70-80% fat, 20-25% protein, and 5-10% carbohydrates.

You must remember that the ratio varies depending on different people thus using an online calculator can greatly help! Make sure that you stick by your macros. The problem with most people is that they tend to eat more protein thinking that protein is always equivalent to fat. Well, not quite. Once you consume protein, the protein will be broken down into a process known as gluconeogenesis and it converts protein into carbs. So, you are back to square one.

To ensure that your body is constantly in the state of ketosis, you need to test the ketone levels in your body to know whether your body is still driving under this state or if you reverted back to your usual glucose-feeding metabolism.

There are several ways to test your body for the presence of ketones. Remember that when your body starts to burn off fats as its main energy source, ketones are spilled over into your blood and urine. And it is even present in you breathe! Since ketones are spilled all over the body, you can test either your urine or breath for its presence. You do not need to punch a tiny hole on your skin for blood testing.

CHAPTER 3:

Foods Included In Keto Diet

Best Foods To Fit Into The Keto Diet For Older Adults

I will go over what food you should consider incorporating into your keto diet. But the general guideline is that all foods that are nutritious and low in carbs are excellent options.

Avocados

Avocados are so famous nowadays in the health community that people associate the word "health" to avocados. This is for a very good reason because avocados are very healthy. They pack lots of vitamins and minerals such as potassium. Moreover, avocados are shown to help the body go into ketosis faster.

Berries

Many fruits pack too many carbs that make them unsuitable in a keto diet, but not berries. They are low in carbs and high in fiber. Some of the best berries to include in your diet are blackberries, blueberries, raspberries, and strawberries.

Butter and Cream

These two food items pack plenty of fat and a very small amount of carbs, making them a good option to include in your keto diet.

Cheese

Milk is not okay. You can get away with cheese though. Cheese is delicious and nutritious. Thankfully, although there are hundreds of types of cheese out there, all of them are low in carbs and full of fat. Eating cheese may even help your muscles and slow down aging.

Coconut Oil

Coconut oil and other coconut-related products such as coconut milk and coconut powder are perfect for a keto diet. Coconut oil, especially, contain MCTs that are converted into ketones by the liver to be used as an immediate source of energy.

Dark Chocolate and Cocoa Powder

These two food items are delicious and contain antioxidants. Dark chocolate is associated with the reduction of heart disease risk by lowering the blood pressure. Just make sure that you choose only dark chocolate with at least 70% cocoa solids.

Eggs

Eggs form the bulk of most food you will eat in a keto diet because they are the healthiest and most versatile food item of them all. Even a large egg contains so little carbs but packs plenty of protein, making it a perfect option for a keto diet.

Moreover, eggs are shown to have an appetite suppression effect, making you feel full for longer as well as regulating blood sugar levels. This leads to lower calorie intake for about a day. Just make sure to eat the entire egg because the nutrients are in the yolk.

Meat and Poultry

KETO FOR WOMEN OVER 50:

These two are the staple food in most keto diets. Most of the keto meals revolve around using these two ingredients. This is because they contain no carbs and pack plenty of vitamins and minerals. Moreover, they are a great source of protein.

Nuts and Seeds

These are also low in carbs but rich in fat. They are also healthy and have a lot of nutrients and fiber. They help reduce heart disease, cancer, depression, and other risks of diseases. The fiber in these also help make you feel full for longer, so you would consume fewer calories and your body would spend more calories digesting them.

Olive Oil

Olive oil is very beneficial for your heart because it contains oleic acid that helps decrease heart disease risk factors. Extra-virgin olive oil is also rich in antioxidants. The best thing is that olive oil can be used as a main source of fat and it has no carbs. The same goes for olive.

Plain Greek Yogurt And Cottage Cheese

These two food items are rich in protein and a small number of carbs, small enough that you can safely include them into your keto diet. They also help suppress your appetite by making you feel full for longer and they can be eaten alone and are still delicious.

Seafood

Fishes and shellfishes are perfect for keto diets. Many fishes are rich in B vitamins, potassium, as well as selenium. Salmon, sardines, mackerel, and other fatty fish also pack a lot of omega-3 fats that help in regulating insulin levels. These are so low in carbs that it is negligible.

Shellfishes are a different story because some contain very few carbs whereas others pack plenty. Shrimps and most crabs are okay but beware of other types of shellfish.

Shirataki Noodles

If you love noodles and pasta but don't want to give up on them, then shirataki noodles are the perfect alternative. They are rich in water content and pack a lot of fiber, so that means low carbs and calories and hunger suppression.

Unsweetened Coffee and Tea

These two drinks are carb-free, so long as you don't add sugar, milk, or any other sweeteners. Both contain caffeine that improves your metabolism and suppresses your appetite. A word of warning to those who love light coffee and tea lattes, though. They are made with non-fat milk and contain a lot of carbs.

Vegetables

Most vegetables pack a lot of nutrients that your body can greatly benefit from even though they are low in calories and carbs. Plus, some of them contain fiber, which helps with your bowel movement. Moreover, your body spends more energy breaking down and digesting food rich in fiber, so it helps with weight loss as well.

Allowed Product List

If you've decided to go on Keto after 50, be sure you won't regret your choice! So when you start something new, the first and the main thing you need to do is consult the Keto dietary features. But most importantly, you must look at the list of allowed products to remember this list and adhere strictly to it.

Don't worry! The low-carb eating plan isn't overly limited. Check out what products you can and must buy in the supermarket and start a new phase in your life.

Meat and Poultry

Chicken, beef, pork, lamb, turkey, veal include no carb, but high protein and fat intake. That is the primary reason why meat and poultry products are known as the staples for the Ketogenic diet. Besides this, bacon and organ meats are also allowed for consumption.

Seafood

When it comes to seafood, you also have an excellent list. You can buy and cook a lot of delicious dishes from:

- Lobster

- Mussels

- Octopus

- Oysters

- Salmon

- Scallops

- Shrimp

- Squid

- Tuna

The most useful Keto seafood is the crab and shrimp. They don't contain carbohydrates at all.

Vegetables

Only low-carb and non-starchy veggies can be eaten by the people who go on the Keto diet. This means that you can add the following vegetables:

- Avocados

- Asparagus

- Bell peppers

- Brussel sprouts

- Celery

- Cucumbers

- Eggplant

- Herbs

- Kale

- Kohlrabi

- Lettuce

- Mushrooms

- Mustard

- Radishes

- Spinach

- Tomatoes

- Zucchini

Dairy Products

You should be careful with dairy. Not all dairy food can be useful for you if you want to stick to the Keto diet. Here are the products you can buy and cook:

- Butter and ghee

- Cottage cheese

- Eggs

- Hard, semi-hard, soft, and cream cheeses

- Heavy cream and whipping cream

- Sour cream

- Unflavored Greek yogurt

Berries

Unfortunately, most fruits have high levels of carbs and can't be included on the Keto diet. However, you can consume:

- Blackberries

- Blueberries

- Raspberries

- Strawberries

Nuts and Seeds

A lot of experts recommend paying attention to nuts and seeds that are high-fat and low-carb. You can add such nuts and seeds to your dishes as:

- Almond

- Brazil nuts

- Chia seeds

- Flaxseed

- Hazelnuts

- Pecans

- Pumpkin seeds

- Walnuts

- Sesame seeds

Coconut and Olive Oils

To cook tasty fatty dishes, you need oil. Coconut and olive oils have unique properties that make them suitable for a Keto diet. These oils are rich in fat and boost ketone production. Moreover, they can be used for salad dressing and adding to cooked dishes.

Low-Carb Drinks

The Keto diet means that you should drink only unsweetened coffee and tea because they don't include carbs and fasten metabolism. Besides, you can drink dark chocolate and cocoa. Such drinks have low levels of carbohydrates and that's why they're permitted.

Prohibited Product List

When it comes to the lists of foods you should avoid on the low-carb, high-fat diet, be attentive and check it carefully. Well, you can't eat:

- Grains (like oatmeal, pasta, bulgur, corn, wheat, buckwheat, rice, etc.)

- Low-fat dairy (fat-free yogurt, skim milk, skim Mozzarella, etc.)

- Most fruits (melon, watermelon, apples, peaches, bananas, grapes, oranges, plums, grapefruits, mangos, cherries, pineapples, pears, etc.)

- Starchy veggies (potatoes, beets, turnips, parsnips, etc.)

- Grain foods (pasta, popcorn, muesli, cereal, bagels, bread, etc.)

- Some oils (soya bean oil, grapeseed oil, sunflower oil, peanut oil, canola oil)

- Typical snack foods (crackers, potato chips, etc.)

- Trans fats (margarine)

- Sweets (candies, buns, pastries, cakes, chocolate, puddings, cookies)

- Sweeteners and added sugars (corn syrup, cane sugar, honey, agave nectar, etc.)

- Sweetened drinks (sweetened coffee and tea, juice, soda, smoothies)

- Alcohol (sweet wines, cider, beer, etc.)

CHAPTER 4:

Introducing You To Keto

How It Works For Your Body

Low-carb diets are known to be among the most controversial eating plans, and the Ketogenic diet is no exception. There is a lot of hype involving this restrictive lifestyle, so it is only natural to wonder whether taking the plunge will be a good choice for your body and overall health. And researching this subject online doesn't help either. Stumbling upon many conflicting theories and contradicting testimonies, you will see that some people (and studies) say how this isn't a good option for a long-term healthy lifestyle, while others (and other studies as well) will try to lure you into ditching the carbs with incredible body transformations, health-improvement stories, and tangible scientific evidence. So, who should you believe? Actually, both!

The thing about the Ketogenic diet is that it isn't a cookie-cutter type of diet, so it is unrealistic to expect that the same meal plan will benefit every type of person, every single body composition, and everyone's unique needs. People can fail for various reasons – they can eat too many carbs without noticing, they can set the wrong macro ratio, or they can even have an underlying condition that will reverse every Ketogenic progress. Others, who manage to do these things right and find the ideal macronutrient ratio, know how to listen to their bodies and consume the food accordingly, can be successful and rewarded Keto dieters for life.

And yes, women over 50 can achieve the latter! With a little bit of discipline and the right eating plan, you can easily get rid of the unpleasant menopause and post-menopause symptoms, and reverse the physical and emotional age-related changes that you struggle with. And the Ketogenic diet can help you with all that.

So, why choose the Ketogenic diet, the question remains. And the answer is pretty simple, actually. Carbohydrates are the biggest enemy for women over 50 because they only worsen the unpleasant symptoms and make the natural transition even harder and more severe. Getting rid of them and embarking on the Keto train will help you restore your health. Besides, the main benefits of the Keto diet are the senior's women's biggest struggles, so there's that.

Influences Of Following The Keto Diet

Keto Improves Your Mood

Unstable mood swings that result in anxiety and/or depression are common among women over 50. These annoying shifts of the emotional state happen as a result of the decrease in estrogen. In the region of our brains, there are estrogen receptors called Medial Amygdala, whose job is to keep the endocrine, stress, and mood, regulated. Once the estrogen levels drop, these receptors fail to do their job properly, and mood swings and mental distress become a usual occurrence.

When we consume a normal, carb-loaded diet, we support rapid changes in our blood sugar levels. And rapid changes in the blood sugar cause women to rapidly change the way in which they feel and behave.

The Ketogenic diet, on the other hand, does the complete opposite. It regulates the blood sugar and slows down this entire process, which ends up delivering stable energy to the brain, which further leads to mood improvement.

Keto Lowers Inflammation

One of the biggest downsides of entering menopause (and getting out of it, as the symptoms mainly continue to live on) is the fact that, during these years, chronic inflammation increases. And since inflammation is the number one culprit for most chronic diseases, it is more than clear how reducing this hazard is your only ticket to better health. Thankfully, the Ketogenic diet can help you achieve just that.

By reducing the carbohydrate intake significantly, a lot of changes start to happen in your body. Stabilizing the blood glucose levels is the most obvious one. Once your blood sugar levels are kept in check and the insulin sensitivity is normalized, your body also decreases the production of free radicals. When that happens, the mitochondria (your cells' powerhouses for energy) starts to produce more of the ATP (Adenosine Triphosphate) molecule, which is in charge of carrying energy.

That being said, the Keto diet plays an important part in creating stronger and healthier mitochondria. When that happens, your body can heal better and can also alleviate diseases effectively. All in all, this process helps your body function better, and support the optimal production of energy, which decreases your chances of developing a chronic and metabolic disease.

But that's not all. Utilizing ketones for energy, instead of glucose, will also decrease neurological inflammation. Once in ketosis, your body will stimulate the Brain-Derived Neurotropic Growth Factor (BDNF) and will close the neuro-inflammatory path. By reducing this inflammation in the brain, Keto women over 50 can eliminate their anxieties and may even treat depression.

Keto Helps You Lose (and Maintain) Weight

Gaining extra pounds (especially around the abdomen) and struggling with controlling the weight are common nuisances that menopausal and post-menopausal women have to deal with. As you can already imagine, this age-related problem is also a result of the decline in the estrogen levels.

Once the estrogen drops down, the overall metabolism is slowed down, and the storage of fat is shifted to the abdomen. This can further lead to insulin resistance, accumulation of toxins, and an increased risk of heart disease.

Keto Lowers the Risk of Cognitive Decline and Eliminates Hot Flashes

Estrogen receptors can be found all throughout the female's body, including the brain. Once the estrogen levels drop when women reach a certain age, these receptors will be left susceptible to dysfunctions and more serious diseases.

One of the main functions of the estrogen hormone is to drive glucose to these receptors and fuel the brain with energy. In a normal diet rich in carbohydrates, the estrogen levels are decreased and the brain stops receiving the same amount of energy it used to get during the pre-menopausal years. That means that older women are at a high risk of brain aging and developing Alzheimer's disease.

What Happens If You Decide To Shift To Keto?

When you adapt to the Ketogenic diet, your body doesn't need glucose for energy, but ketones, which means that the loss in estrogen will not be that big of a deal for your brain. Being in ketosis and using ketones will provide the brain cells with steady energy to the brain cells. This is what decreases the menopausal and post-menopausal symptoms such as hot flashes and brain fog.

Besides the formerly mentioned benefits that are especially important for women over 50, choosing to go Keto will reward senior women with many different positive changes as well:

- The triglyceride levels can drop drastically

- The good HDL cholesterol will be increased

- High blood pressure can be lowered

- The symptoms of Parkinson's disease will be significantly reduced

- Lower heartburn and support gut health

- Get rid of oily skin

-   Help regulate the polycystic ovary syndrome

-   Will get rid of oxidative stress and may increase the lifespan

But what if you are not that affected by the menopausal symptoms and you believe you are in a pretty good physical and emotional state? No hot flashes, no anxiety… Nothing that indicates you have reached a certain milestone. How to know if you can benefit from the Ketogenic diet if you are not that attuned to your body?

Your body sends you signals constantly. And even if you do not recognize them, or if they are not severe and don't come in the form of pain or discomfort, they are there.

Below you will find a list of symptoms in which your body tells you it needs – and will benefit from – more fat. If you see recognize yourself in at least two of them, then you should definitely give the Keto diet a try:

-   You get bloated after meals or have a "food pregnancy" most of the days

-   You have more weight than you should

-   You have a headache most days

-   You are constipated or feel sluggish pretty much every day

-   20-30 minutes after eating you feel extremely tired and sleepy

-   You struggle to focus and find crowded places extremely overwhelming

-   Your skin flakes

-   You gain weight even though you are mindful of your bites

-   You just cannot quit sugar

- You are sensitive to some foods that you haven't had reactions to before

- You are always hungry

- You need regular pick-me-ups in the afternoon or you cannot function the rest of the day

- You feel wonky and tired on a regular basis

- Your joints hurt in the morning and/or after meals

- You are dependent on vitamin supplements, which your doctor has prescribed

- Your hair has been frizzy recently

CHAPTER 5:

Benefits Of Keto Diet

The keto diet has become so popular in recent years because of the success people have noticed. Not only have they managed to lose weight, but scientific studies show that the keto diet can help you improve your health in many others. As when starting any new diet or exercise routine, there may seem to be some disadvantages so we will go over those for the keto diet as well. But most people agree that the benefits outweigh the adjustment period!

Helps You Lose Weight

For most people, this is the first and foremost benefit of switching to keto! Their former diet method may have stalled for them or they were starting to notice weight creeping back on. With keto, studies have shown that people have been able to follow this diet and relay fewer hunger pangs and suppressed appetite while losing weight at the same time! You are minimizing your carbohydrate intake which means less blood sugar spikes. Often, those fluctuations in blood sugar levels are what make you feel hungrier and more prone to snacking in between meals. Instead, by guiding the body towards ketosis, you are eating a more fulfilling diet of fat and protein and harnessing energy from ketone molecules instead of glucose. Studies show that low carb diets are very effective in reducing visceral fat (the type of fat you commonly see around the abdomen that increases as you become overweight and obese). This reduces your risk of obesity and improves your health in the long run.

Decreases The Risk Of Type 2 Diabetes.

The problem with carbohydrates is how unstable they make blood sugar levels. This can be very dangerous for people who have diabetes or are considered pre-diabetic due to unstable blood sugar levels or family history. Keto is a great option because of the minimal intake of carbohydrates it requires. Instead, you are harnessing the majority of your calories from fat or protein which will not cause blood sugar spikes and ultimately put less pressure on the pancreas to secrete insulin. Many studies have found that diabetes patients who followed the keto diet lost more weight and ultimately reduced their fasting glucose levels. This is great news for patients who have unstable blood sugar levels or are hoping to avoid or reduce their diabetes medication intake.

Improve Cardiovascular Risk Symptoms To Overall Lower Your Chances Of Having Heart Disease.

Most people assume that following keto that is so high in fat content has to increase your risk of coronary heart disease or heart attack. But the research proves otherwise! Research shows that switching to keto can lower your blood pressure, increase your HDL good cholesterol, and reduce your triglyceride fatty acid levels. That's because the fats you are consuming on keto are healthy and high-quality fats so they tend to reverse many unhealthy symptoms of heart disease. They boost your "good" HDL cholesterol numbers and decrease your "bad" LDL cholesterol numbers. It also decreases the level of triglyceride fatty acids in the bloodstream. A high level of these can lead to stroke, heart attack, or premature death. And what are the high levels of fatty acids linked to? High consumption of carbohydrates. With the keto diet, you are drastically cutting your intake of carbohydrates to improve fatty acid levels and improve other risk factors. A 2018 study on the keto diet found that it can improve as many as 22 out of 26 risk factors for cardiovascular heart disease! These factors can be very important to some people, especially those who have a history of heart disease in their family.

Increases The Body's Energy Levels.

We compared briefly the difference between the glucose molecules synthesized from a high carbohydrates intake versus ketones produced on the keto diet. Ketones are made by the liver and use fat molecules you already have stored. This makes them much more energy-rich and a lasting source of fuel compared to glucose, a simple sugar molecule. These ketones can give you a burst of energy physically as well as mentally allow you to have greater focus, clarity, and attention to detail.

Decreases Inflammation In The Body

Inflammation on its own is a natural response by the body's immune system, but when it becomes uncontrollable, it can lead to an array of health problems, some severe, some minor. The many health concerns include acne, autoimmune conditions, arthritis, psoriasis, irritable bowel syndrome, and even acne and eczema. Often, removing sugars and carbohydrates from your diet can help patients of these diseases avoid flare-ups - and the good news is keto does just that! A 2008 research study found that keto decreased a blood marker linked to high inflammation in the body by nearly 40%. This is great news for people who may suffer from an inflammatory disease and are willing to change their diet to hopefully see improvement.

Increases Your Mental Functioning Level

Like we elaborated earlier, the energy-rich ketones can boost the body's physical and mental levels of alertness. Research has shown that keto is a much better energy source for the brain than simple sugar glucose molecules are. With nearly 75% of your diet coming from healthy fats, the brain's neural cells and mitochondria have a better source of energy to be able to function at the highest level. Some studies have tested patients on the keto diet and found they had higher cognitive functioning, better memory recall, and were less susceptible to memory loss. The keto diet can even decrease the occurrence of migraines which can be very detrimental to patients.

Decreases Risk Of Diseases Like Alzheimer's, Parkinson's, And Epilepsy.

The keto diet was actually created in the 1920s as a way to combat epilepsy in children. From there, research has found that keto can improve your cognitive functioning level and protect brain cells from injury or damage. This is very good to reduce the risk of neurodegenerative disease which begins in the brain due to neural cells mutating and functioning with damaged parts or lower than peak optimal functioning. Studies have found that following keto can improve the mental functioning of patients who suffer from diseases like Alzheimer's or Parkinson's. These neurodegenerative diseases sadly have no cure, but the keto diet could improve symptoms as they progress. Researchers believe that is due to cutting out carbs from your diet which reduces the occurrence of blood sugar spikes that the body's neural cells have to continually adjust to.

Can Regulate Hormones In Women Who Have Pcos And Pms

Women who have PCOS (polycystic ovary syndrome) suffer from infertility which can be very heartbreaking for young couples trying to start a family. There is no cure for this condition, but it is believed that it is related to many similar diabetic symptoms like obesity and high insulin levels. This causes the body to produce more sex hormones which can lead to infertility. The keto diet has become a popular method to try and regulate insulin and hormone levels and could increase a woman's chances of getting pregnant.

Disadvantages

Your body will have an adjustment period. It depends from person to person on how many days that will be, but when you start any new diet or exercise routine, your body has to adjust to the new normal. With the keto diet, you are drastically cutting your carbohydrates intake, so the body has to adjust to that. You may feel slow, weak, fatigued, and like you are not thinking as quick or fast as you used to. It just means your body is adjusting to keto and once this adjustment period is done, you will see the weight loss results you anticipated.

If you are an athlete, you may need more carbohydrates. If you still want to try keto as an athlete, it's important you talk to your nutritionist or trainer to see how the diet can be tweaked for you. Most athletes require a greater intake of carbs than the keto diet requires which means they may have to up their intake in order to assure they have the energy for their training sessions. High endurance sports (like rugby or soccer) and heavy weightlifting do require a greater intake of carbohydrates. If you're an athlete wanting to follow keto and gain the health benefits, it's important you first talk to your trainer before making any changes to your diet.

You have to carefully count your daily macros! For beginners, this can be tough, and even people already on keto can become lazy about this. People are often used to eating what they want without worrying about just how many grams of protein or carbs it contains. With keto, you have to be meticulous about counting your intake to ensure you are maintaining the necessary keto breakdown (75% fat, 20% protein, ~5% carbs). The closer you stick to this, the better results you will see regarding weight loss and other health benefits. If your weight loss has stalled or you're not feeling as energetic as you hoped, it could be because your macros are off. Find a free calorie counting app that and be sure you look at the ingredients of everything you're eating and cooking.

CHAPTER 6:

How Age Affects The Ketogenic Diet

Nutrition is vital to maintain health and to lead an active and fulfilling life. There is another fact that your nutritional need changes throughout your life and that's why eating healthy becomes more important. If you are eating unhealthy food and suffering from nutritional deficiencies, then this will bring harmful outcomes, and you will lead a poor-quality life.

Childhood: In the initial years of life, the little bodies need essential nutrients along with regular nutrients to ensure they develop and grow physically and mentally. The food should provide high energy to support the rapid growth of bodies at this age. Also, childhood is the time of learning and experiencing new foods and developing taste and smell sense, which shape their eating habits for later in life. Therefore, children should be encouraged to consume a variety of foods every day. The key nutrient in children's diet includes protein which is necessary for growth, calcium and vitamin D to grow strong bones. Adolescence: The body around this time goes through significant emotional and physical changes due to puberty. Moreover, maturing sexuality increases the muscles growth and strengthens the bones, and this is a perfect opportunity for children to build strong bones for later. For this reason, it is really essential that the body meets its calcium requirement. For this, dairy milk products are perfect healthy choices such as yogurt, milk, and cheese that are well known for high-quality protein and calcium-rich sources. Iron is an also essential bone nutrient that can be obtained from red meat, chicken, kidney beans, spinach, and mussels.

Encourage them to have water or milk as beverages and healthy snacks to combat craving and untimely hunger. Also, make-ahead some smoothies, prepare grab-and-go food options like toasts and sandwiches and do meal prepping for children that can't sit long enough to eat food at the meal table.

Adulthood: This is the time when you have to focus on maintaining the healthy body you have developed through your childhood and adolescence. Therefore, the body should get good enough nutrition like protein, calcium, vitamins, and phosphorus that helps you stay active, energetic and maintain bones and muscles that tend to decrease as we move forward in age. Focus on eating healthy foods that give you all the nutrients, which make you feel great without disturbing your ideal body weight and reduce the factors of ailments like diabetes and heart diseases.

Older age: At the old age, the body needs the same or even more protein, minerals, and vitamins. For example, after the age of 50, your body's ability to absorb specific vitamins fades due to hormonal changes, and you don't have enough stomach acid to break down food sources. So, if you aren't eating foods that don't have these vitamins or not taking nutrients supplements then you may suffer from dangerous ailments. Also, you may eat less than earlier due to reduced appetite, health issues or medications. In that case, eat little and often can effectively help your body in getting essential nutrients that support mobility, active mind, growth, mental and physical performance. Enjoy a variety of foods and drinks and go for nutritious and natural options for foods that contain a range of nutrients. Similarly, you may not notice thirst in your later years, but keeping your body hydrated is important at any age. With these examples, you have to make little bits of changes in what you eat and drink to achieve optimal health no matter what your age is.

There are many scientific theories out there that explain how the human body ages and deteriorates over time, two of which are a free radical theory of aging and glycation theory of aging.

The free radical theory explains that our body becomes damaged because of the free radicals trying to bind to the molecules in our body in their search for more electron, which leads to damage and inflammation. In the process of binding, your molecule becomes unstable and binds with your other molecule to get its electron, and the cycle repeats in a process known as oxidation, causing a lot of damage over time. The solution this theory proposed is to increase your body's pool of antioxidants

KETO FOR WOMEN OVER 50:

because they have an extra electron to give to the free radicals in your body, thus preventing them from taking and destabilizing your body's molecules.

The glycation theory of aging proposes that we age because of the glycation damage from high blood sugar. That means the excess sugar in the body clings onto the proteins in the body, preventing them from doing their jobs, which can lead to many complications, one of which is diabetes.

But how does the keto diet come in? Keto diets can help the body slow the aging process in many ways:

1. Keto diet minimizes damages done by oxidation and increases the body's store of uric acid and other antioxidants.

2. Ketosis increases the mitochondrial glutathione, which is a potent antioxidant that resides within the mitochondria, the powerhouse of your cell. Antioxidants that are digested orally are not very effective in protecting your cells. But ketosis supports the cell directly.

3. Keto diets are very low in sugar, meaning that your blood sugar level would be much lower, reducing the chance of glycation damages.

4. Keto diets are low in carbs, which improves blood sugar control level and suppress appetite because they have the same effects as fasting.

5. Keto diets also reduce triglycerides, which are the fatty acids in the bloodstream that are used to measure heart disease risk. You want triglycerides in your body to be as low as possible.

In short, keto diets reduce your blood sugar level, prevent glycation damages, and inflammation. These three conditions are associated with all sorts of diseases that lead to death. Therefore, keto diets ate the best way to reduce blood sugar and insulin levels, increase your longevity and well-being.

38 | P a g e

CHAPTER 7:

Women Over 50 And Ketogenic Diet

Getting to the age of 50 means many physical and psychological changes in women such as menopause, hormonal problems, inflammation, irritability, weak muscles and bones, lethargy, and the list goes on. Some women develop diabetes, Alzheimer's, and cardiovascular problems as well.

Why A Normal Keto Diet Is Not Recommended For Women Over 50

With a normal Keto diet, you cut your carbs down to minimum levels, i.e. less than 15 grams. Cutting down carbs severely and suddenly is bad for you because due to ageing your metabolism decreases by 25%, and with every passing year, your bones and muscles become weaker and weaker.

We also become more vulnerable to many physiological and psychological diseases, such as cardiovascular disease, obesity, Alzheimer's, or diabetes. Adopting a regular Keto diet plan can result in many side effects, such as:

- Headaches

- Dizziness

- Fatigue

- Brain fog and difficulty focusing

- Lack of motivation and irritability

- Nausea

- Keto flue

- Inflammation

And more.

These side effects cause many women to pull back and lose hope. It's all because you haven't been told before about the likely side effects that you can suffer if you dive head first into the Keto diet. However, consuming the right amount of fats while eating as much as you desire within the range of the specific foods presented in this book, you will get your desired results.

For this, you need a specific Keto diet plan which will not only benefit you via weight loss but will also help build muscles, stabilizes your blood sugar levels, and maximize your energy levels. And for all this, the Keto diet for women over 50 is a perfect option for you.

How The Ketogenic Diet Can Aid With The Signs And Symptoms Of Ageing And Menopause

For ageing women, menopause will bring severe changes and challenges, but the ketogenic diet can help you switch gears effortlessly to continue enjoying a healthy and happy life. Menopause can upset hormonal levels in women, which consequently affects brainpower and cognitive abilities. Furthermore, due to less production of estrogens and progesterone, your sex drive declines, and you suffer from sleep issues and mood problems. Let's have a look at how a ketogenic diet will help solve these side effects.

Enhanced Cognitive Functions

Usually, hormone estrogen ensures the continuous flow of glucose into your brain. But after menopause, the estrogen levels begin to drop dramatically, so does the amount of glucose reaching the bran. As a result, your functional brainpower will start to deteriorate. However, by following the

KETO FOR WOMEN OVER 50:

keto diet for women over 50, the problem of glucose intake is circumvented. This results in enhanced cognitive functions and brain activity.

Hormonal Balance

Usually, women face major symptoms of menopause due to hormonal imbalances. The keto diet for women over 50 works by stabilizing these imbalances such as estrogen. This aids in experiencing fewer and bearable menopausal symptoms like hot flashes. The keto diet also balances blood sugar levels and insulin and helps in controlling insulin sensitivity.

Intensified Sex Drive

The keto diet surges the absorption of vitamin D, which is essential for enhancing sex drive. Vitamin D ensures stable levels of testosterone and other sex hormones that could become unstable due to low levels of testosterone.

Better Sleep

Glucose disturbs your blood sugar levels dramatically, which in turn leads to poor quality of sleep. Along with other menopausal symptoms, good sleep becomes a huge problem as you age. The keto diet for women over 50 not only balances blood glucose levels, but also stabilizes other hormones like cortisol, melatonin, and serotonin warranting an improved and better sleep.

Reduces inflammation

Menopause can upsurge the inflammation levels by letting potential harmful invaders in our system, which result in uncomfortable and painful symptoms. Keto diet for women over 50 uses the healthy anti-inflammatory fats to reduce inflammation and lower pain in your joints and bones.

Fuel your brain

Are you aware that your brain is composed of 60% fat or more? This infers that it needs a larger amount of fat to keep it functioning optimally. In other words, the ketones from the keto diet serve as the energy source that fuels your brain cells.

Nutrient deficiencies

Ageing women tend to have higher deficiencies in essential nutrients such as, iron deficiency which leads to brain fog and fatigue; Vitamin B12 deficiency, which leads to neurological conditions like dementia; Fats deficiency, that can lead to problems with cognition, skin, vision; and Vitamin D deficiency that not only causes cognitive impairment in older adults and increase the risk of heart disease but also contribute to the risk of developing cancer. On a keto diet, the high-quality proteins ensure adequate and excellent sources of these important nutrients.

Controlling Blood Sugar

Research has suggested a link between poor blood sugar levels and brain diseases such as Alzheimer's disease, Parkinson's Disease, or Dementia. Some factors contributing to Alzheimer's disease may include:

- Enormous intake of carbohydrates, especially from fructose—which is drastically reduced in the ketogenic diet.

- Lack of nutritional fats and good cholesterol — which are copious and healthy in the keto diet

Keto diet helps control blood sugar and improve nutrition; which in turn not only improves insulin response and resistance but also protects against memory loss which is often a part of ageing.

CHAPTER 8:

How Is Weight Loss Achieved On Ketogenic Diets For Women Over 50?

Now that we've gone over the ketogenic diet and all the things involved with being on the ketogenic diet, it is a good time to look at some tips and tips and tricks to being successful on the keto diet.

Limit Your Carbohydrate Intake

The whole point of the ketogenic diet is to substantially reduce your consumption of carbohydrates. Even if practicing a gentler keto, as recommended for women over 50, you still need to be mindful of the carbs you are consuming. Be sure not to eat hidden carbohydrates that are often found in processed foods. Be wary of "lite" and "low fat" foods. They often get their flavor from sugar. Sugar is, of course, low in fat. On the contrary, sugar is high in carbohydrates. It is a good idea to eliminate almost all forms of sugar on the ketogenic diet. Don't let your carb intake exceed 10%.

Introduce Coconut Oil Into Your Diet

Coconut oil is full of nutrients that metabolize quickly in your liver and is converted to energy right away. Consuming coconut oil may help you reach ketosis faster. It's a really easy way to motivate your body to be in ketosis.

Exercise

It is important to maintain your muscle mass, perhaps increase your muscle mass. Make sure that you're doing exercises involving strength and endurance. Keep the exercises a low-intensity level so that you're burning fat, and not using carbohydrates.

Eat Enough Fat.

You have to be sure, while you are on the ketogenic diet, that you are eating enough fat. The fat you eat is going to be converted into energy. You need to have enough fat in your body to supply energy to your brain, organs, and muscles to sustain yourself and your activities. Additionally, make sure that you are using your macros to decide what to eat, and that you recalculate your macros from time to time. Be sure you know what you're eating and that you're meeting your nutrient needs, including fat, for each day.

Track Your Food

Keep a record of your food consumption. Be sure to add in all the "bits and bites" that pass your lips. You know, the food that you test while cooking? That corner of a cookie you broke off as a little nibble? Record everything you eat so that you know you're meeting your macros. Read labels to make sure you know what you're eating. This book will include a guide on raw foods and meats so that you can calculate how many nutrients are in the foods that you are eating after you have eliminated processed foods from your diet.

Drink Lots Of Water

Water is essential to the body, and you will lose a lot of water on the ketogenic diet. The water must be replaced, especially after exercise. You may also want to take a mineral supplement or drink water with electrolytes so that your chemical balance is maintained after working out. Replacing the water lost through sweat and urination will keep your body working properly. You will feel better if you stay hydrated throughout your ketogenic diet.

Reduce Your Stress

Try to remain stress-free during your ketogenic diet. As mentioned, cortisol levels in your body will cause your body to retain fat, especially in the abdominal region. You want to be sure that your body is not working at cross purposes. Stress may trigger your body to store fat in reaction to stress while you are trying to lose fat on your ketogenic diet. Make sure you incorporate activities in your day to reduce your stress level. Some people find yoga is a good way to relax. Others use hobbies as a way to relieve tension and reduce stress.

Get Lots Of Sleep

Make sure you get enough sleep. Each night your body needs 7 to 9 hours of sleep. Sleep allows us time to rejuvenate our bodies and store up energy. Be sure to do things that promote a sleep-inducing atmosphere. Turn off the lights, limit the use of electronics and like computers and smartphones within 30 minutes of sleeping and refrain from using them in bed. Turn off the television and prepare your room and your body for sleep. Try to maintain a consistent schedule of sleep. These things may make it easier to get to sleep. People on the keto diet have reported better sleep, reduced snoring, and waking up refreshed. Set the scene so that you will be able to benefit from better sleep on the diet.

Know Your Goals

Before you start the ketogenic diet, determine your goals, and write down the reasons why you're on the ketogenic diet. If you want to lose weight, also note why you want to lose weight. This is important, so you can always refer back to the reasons you began the diet. It is sometimes helpful to remember what your goals are and why you want to meet those goals. This will be a good touchstone when you want to reach for a cookie or a sugary drink. Make sure you have that goal handy so that when you're feeling weak, you can remind yourself of your goals are and be determined to stick to them.

CHAPTER 9:

Calories And Macros Intake For Losing Weight

Macronutrients are found in all food products. These are nutrients that nourish the body. Carbohydrates, proteins, and fats are contained in the calories consumed and should be monitored during the ketone diet. The necessary information can be found on the nutritional label of foods. Measure individual portions carefully to ensure you have accurate nutritional information. These nutrients that are tracked are usually called "macro," which is an abbreviated version of the word macro elements. This book specifies the macros you need to know to get a ketogenic diet plan. By modifying SKD and HPKD, you can create a more fluid keto plan to meet the needs of women over 50. We will first analyze the carbohydrates. These will be net carbohydrates. The net gram of carbs is determined by subtracting grams of dietary fiber and grams of sugar alcohol from the total number of carbs. Dietary fiber does not release insulin into the body. The same goes for sugar alcohols. As a result, you can eat more nutrient-dense foods and satisfy your thirst and hunger. Then we will see the fats. You will eat 60 to 75% of your food as fat. This allows you to include a wide range of products in the diet, such as bacon and pork skins. Avocados, nuts, and other foods will be included on the menu. As you will eat unprocessed foods, it is essential to eat healthy fats, including oil from natural food sources, such as avocado oil and coconut oil. High-quality butter and clarified butter will also be a good source of fat. When we start thinking about protein doesn't have to be lean meat. The keto protein does not have to be thin but must contain a lot of fat to consume the right amount of fat. A ketogenic diet is only valid if you eat a lot of fat. Now let's start the macro calculation. To calculate the gram of net carbohydrates that will be included in your daily diet, it is essential to determine your body weight and, therefore, your body fat percentage. To do this, weigh yourself. After determining the weight, divide the body weight by the height in inches and the height of the square in square inches. Multiply by 703, and you will get a body mass index or a body mass index.

For Example:

Lbs / height in inches, square, 703 = BMI.

So really, if you're a woman 5 feet 6 inches long and weighs 200 pounds, it's 200 / 66² x 703 = 32.28.

The BMI is 32.28.

Then calculate your body fat percentage. (1.2 x BMI) + (0.23 * age) - 5.4 is the percentage of body fat.

When we combine the BMI from our female example,

(1.2 * 32.28) + (0.23 * 55) - 5.4 = 45.98

The percentage of body fat is therefore 45.98%.

Now that you have a body fat percentage take your body fat percentage and multiply it by your body weight. 45.98% x 200 pounds

This corresponds to 91.96 pounds of body fat. Subtract body fat from body mass, and you will get LBM (lean mass).

So 200 - 91.96 is equal to 108.04. LBM is 108.04.

It's time to determine how many macronutrients you need to eat each day. We can start by calculating the protein.

Its 0.8 grams per kilogram of lean body mass.

In our example, 0.8 * 108.04 is equal to 84 grams.

This equals 346 calories because each gram of protein contains four calories.

In our example, 20% of the calories per day come from proteins. Therefore, 346 calories / 0.20 is 1,730 calories per day.

The total number of calories is 1,730 calories per day.

To determine the number of carbohydrates, let's look at the number of glucose in a milder keto.

10% of your daily calories will come from carbohydrates.

10% of 1,730 calories are 173 calories. If you divide 173 calories into 4 (there are four calories in each sugar), you will get 43.25 g of carbohydrates in a daily quantity. Rest for daily calorie calories: 346 calories, protein 86.50 g 20% + 173 calories, Carbohydrates 43.25 g 10% 519 calories protein and carbohydrates -1730 (total calories)

Fat 134.56 g 70%

These macros will change when your BMI and LBM change. Remember to adapt your macros every 4 to 5 weeks, while losing weight so that the macros are precise. You have to record what you eat and check the success of the weight loss. This will allow you to track how your body reacts to food combinations. Everyone is different, and it's essential to see what it's like to eat different foods and food combinations as you approach ketosis. Remember to eat whole grains and get fiber in green leafy vegetables. You will also be very familiar with nutrition labels to make sure you don't eat hidden carbohydrates without realizing it.

CHAPTER 10:

Specific Fitness Exercises for Women Over 50 to Support the Ketogenic Diet

It is relevant to get all the knowledge necessary on how to exercise while on the keto diet to keep you from running into any problems.

When thinking about excessive weight, the next thing that comes to your mind is probably the amount of food you will have to avoid. In truth, there are also other ways to lose weight. That is the work out which, if combined with a diet, especially the ketogenic one, cannot be improvised in any way.

If you are thinking about going into keto to lose weight, then these questions might come to your mind: Is exercise okay on the keto diet? Can you go ahead with exercising on keto even if you haven't exercised for a long time?

The Benefit Of Exercise On The Keto Diet

Yes, you should exercise while on keto.

To answer the first question of whether exercising is safe while on the keto diet, I say YES. Apart from the fact that exercise has lots of benefits when mixed with keto, it also helps immensely in decreasing the risk of several cardiovascular diseases. It is also excellent for mental health.

The only caution is that you only have to be careful about the types of exercise you choose to do. It might be better if you seek the advice of a doctor, a certified personal trainer, or a nutrition specialist. You just have to make sure you select the best workout routine that goes hand-in-hand with a ketogenic diet.

How Keto Impacts Your Exercise Performance

Your cells produce energy for your body by making use of two primary energy sources, which include fatty acids and glucose. As I said earlier, ketosis is a state where your body uses fatty acids predominantly as a source of energy through a process known as beta-oxidation. When you start dieting, your body makes more use of fatty acid to generate energy. However, this shift takes time for your body to adapt to it.

During this time, the body experiences the keto flu (because of the adjustment period), and sleep and irritability problems may arise. You might be experiencing the keto flu because of the following reasons:

1. Your body needs time to adapt to the keto diet

2. Micronutrients and electrolyte are deficient

3. Withdrawal from carbs that have the same symptoms with caffeine withdrawal occurs

Because of this adaptation time, your exercise plan might be interrupted during the first few weeks - you are going to have a harder time recovering from workouts. The good news here is that while your body adapts to the keto, you can still benefit from exercise at the same time.

Pros Of Exercise In Keto (Health Benefits Of Exercising In Ketosis)

According to certain studies, ketogenic diets could hinder exercise in the long term, but some others have shown that it has lots of benefits. For example, in a recent study of ultra-endurance athletes who went through 3 hours run, it came to fore that athletes who were on a low-carb diet experienced two to three times more loss of fat in 20 months than those on the high carb diet. Muscle recovery has also been shown to be the same for all athletes.

Also, several studies have shown that ketosis helps obese people to maintain blood glucose levels during exercise. Another benefit of ketosis is seen in its ability to help you in not getting tired during long periods of aerobic exercise. It also enables people who perform high-intensity workouts to recover faster.

Top 3 Exercises For Keto Beginners

There are several types of exercises for different stages of intensity. There is the glycolytic short burst exercise that requires the use of glucose as fuel. Activities under this category are usually known as High-Intensity Interval Training (HIIT) and CrossFit-style weight training. As soon as you adapt to the keto diet, you will be able to deal with HIIT training. During the period of adjusting to the keto diet, your body is not ready at all to use ketones for energy.

Exercises suitable for you at this stage are:

Light cardio

Specific aerobic exercises are perfect for you if you are just getting started on keto, although you have to keep them at low intensity (a maximum heart rate of 40-50%). The following cardiovascular workouts can help you ease into keto diet while you adapt to it:

- swimming

- hiking

- rowing

- biking

Simple resistance workouts

Many people often believe that you need carbs to build muscle, but this is not true. It does not matter if you are adapted to keto or not. As far as you eat enough protein, you will be able to build strength and lean mass with ketones serving as fuel. You can try some light weightlifting as you transit into the keto diet.

Flexibility and balance

Flexibility and balance should be part of your exercise routine to avoid injury and increase your motion range. It also activates your core muscles. These exercises include:

- Pilates

- Yoga

- Gymnastics

Do not under-eat before working out

Even though the keto diet is very restrictive, you should ensure that you give your body enough nutrients. Cutting out an entire food group means you are reducing a lot of calories. However, it is important to remember that the keto diet can suppress appetite so that even when you under-eat, you might not feel hungry. Consequently, you might not know you are not giving your body enough nutrition. Combining working out with under-eating will make you feel miserable, and it will affect your performance.

Making keto and exercising a perfect match

If you are just getting started on a keto diet, and you want to engage in some high intensity, it is essential to know the version of the keto diet that is appropriate for you. One of the best things about keto is that it can be modified, depending on your needs. This ability to adapt the keto diet to your needs in combination with your workout routine goes a long way in giving you a healthy life.

CHAPTER 11:

Intermittent Fasting And Keto

What Is Intermittent Fasting?

Much like the Ketogenic Diet, Intermittent Fasting is picking up more popularity by the year! IF is an eating pattern you are going to follow with periods of fasting and periods of eating. When you eat in this manner, you will be focusing on the foods allowed on the ketogenic diet, along with deciding when you are going to eat them.

Fasting has been practiced throughout our entire time on earth. When you think about it, our ancestors did not have food available year-round. When they were unable to find food, they had to learn how to function without food for extended periods of time. In the modern world, we have a McDonald's at every corner, which is both a blessing and a curse! For this reason, fasting is actually much more natural for us compared to eating three or even four meals in a day!

How Does It Work?

If this is your first time trying the Ketogenic Diet, you may want to wait to incorporate this style of eating. It is going to be enough work figuring out what you are allowed to eat on the Ketogenic Diet. When you are ready, there are several types of intermittent fasting that you can try out. Much like with our diets, everyone is allowed to be on a different schedule. What works for you may not work for your friend! But this is one of the best parts of the diet; it is completely customizable to your needs!

- 16/8 Method

This first popular method is known as the Leangains Protocol. For this method, you will skip breakfast and only eat for eight hours during the day. An example of this could be 12-8p.m. Once those hours are up, you would then fast for sixteen hours. During your fast, you eat nothing or very little amounts of food if you are desperate.

- 5:2 Diet

This next method is a bit different compared to typical fasting. For the 5:2 diet, you spend two days eating only 500-600 calories. On the rest of the days, you are allowed to eat normally.

- Eat-Stop-Eat

The Eat-Stop-Eat fasting method involves not eating for 24 hours straight for one or two days a week. For the other days, you are allowed to eat normally.

- Crescendo Method

For women over 50, this may be your best option. For the Crescendo Method, you will only be fasting for 12-16 hours for 2-3 days a week. These days of fasting should be nonconsecutive and spaced throughout your week. For example, you would want to fast for Monday, Wednesday, and again on Friday.

Intermittent fasting works because during these fasts, you are reducing your overall calorie intake for the week. The fewer calories you consume, the more weight you are going to lose. For this reason, you need to make sure you are not compensating for this calorie reduction by overeating during the times you are allowed to eat. It is all about moderation and finding a good balance in your diet.

Intermittent Fasting And Hormones

As you follow the Ketogenic Diet combined with intermittent fasting, there are several things that will be happening to you on a molecular and cellular level. One of the major benefits being that as you fast, your body will adjust your hormone levels to make your body fat more accessible. This is beneficial on the Ketogenic Diet because you are now using the fat as energy, anyway!

Fasting also initiates cellular repair within your body. This process is known as autophagy. During autophagy, your cells begin to digest and remove any dysfunctional proteins that are old and built up inside of your cells. Fasting also helps promote proper gene expression that may help protect against disease and help you live a longer and healthier life!

What's The Benefit For Weight Loss?

If you are looking to lose weight on the Ketogenic Diet, it will be beneficial for you to pair it with Intermittent Fasting. With this manner of eating, you will be eating fewer meals and reducing your number of calories automatically. Once this is complete, your body will begin lowering the insulin in your system and increases the number of fat-burning hormones in your system. This meaning that through short-term fasting, you can increase your metabolic rate and get rid of that excess weight!

Health Benefits Of Intermittent Fasting

While weight loss is an incredible benefit in itself, Intermittent Fasting will offer you several other benefits as well. Some of the other benefits include:

- Decreased Inflammation

- Improved Heart Health

- Increased Brain Health

- Increased Life Spans

Intermittent Fasting can also help lead you to a simpler lifestyle. When you are eating three to four meals a day, this requires a lot of time to cook and plan healthy meals. When you are only eating for a certain amount of time, this gives you more time to do the things that you want without worrying about fitting a meal in!

Is It Dangerous For Women Over 50?

Risks of Intermittent Fasting

With those benefits in mind, it should be stated that Intermittent Fasting is not for everyone. For example, if you are underweight or have a history of eating disorders, you will want to consult with a professional before you begin Intermittent Fasting or the Ketogenic Diet. With these two methods combined, your diet will be doing you more harm than good.

It should be noted that there are also some side-effects you can expect on Intermittent Fasting. One of the major symptoms will be hunger. Up until this point, your body has been used to be provided with food all day long. When you take this away, you will probably get hungry. You may also feel weak at times, but these symptoms should go away once your body adapts to the new schedule.

You will also want to consult with a professional if you have any of the following:

- Pregnant or Breastfeeding

- History of Amenorrhea

- Trying to Get Pregnant

- Take Medications

- Have Low Blood Pressure or Problems with Blood Sugar Regulation

- Have Diabetes

CHAPTER 12:

Breakfast Recipes

Kale Avocado Smoothie

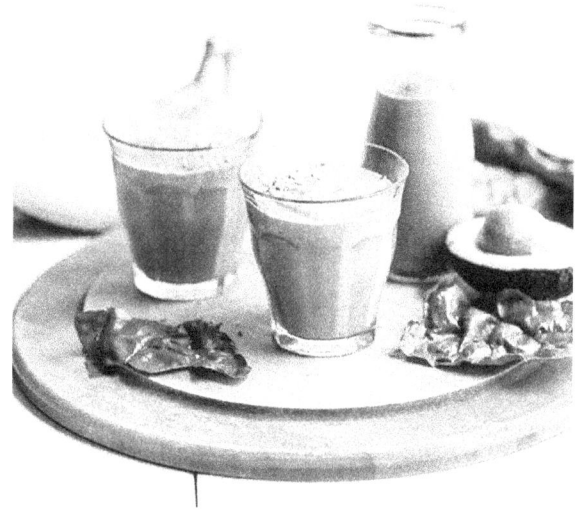

Preparation Time: 5 minutes

Cooking Time: 0 minutes

Servings: 1

Ingredients:

1 cup fresh chopped kale

½ cup chopped avocado

¾ cup unsweetened almond milk

¼ cup full-fat yogurt, plain

3 to 4 ice cubes

1 tablespoon fresh lemon juice

Liquid stevia extract, to taste

Directions:

Combine the kale, avocado, and almond milk in a blender.

Pulse the ingredients several times.

Add the remaining ingredients and blend them until smooth.

Pour into a large glass and enjoy immediately.

Nutrition:

Calories: 250

Fat: 19g

Protein: 6g

Carbs: 17.5g

Fiber: 6.5g

Almond Butter Protein Smoothie

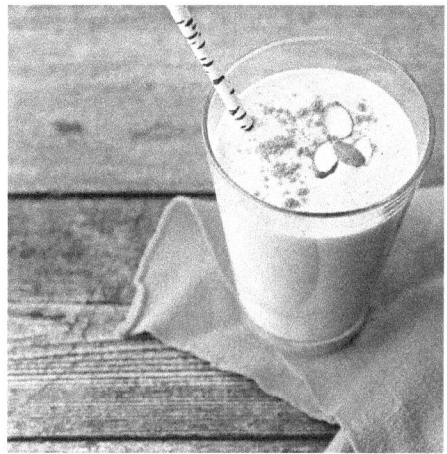

Preparation Time: 5 minutes

Cooking Time: 0 minutes

Servings: 1

Ingredients: 1 cup unsweetened almond milk - ½ cup full-fat yogurt, plain

¼ cup vanilla egg white protein powder - 1 tablespoon almond butter

Pinch ground cinnamon - Liquid stevia extract, to taste

Directions:

In a blender, add the almond milk and yoghurt. Pulse several times over the ingredients. Stir in the remaining ingredients and blend until smooth. Pour into a big glass, and instantly enjoy it.

Nutrition:

Calories: 315 -Fat: 16.5g - Protein: 31.5g - Carbohydrates: 12g - Sugar: 2.5g

Almond Butter Muffins

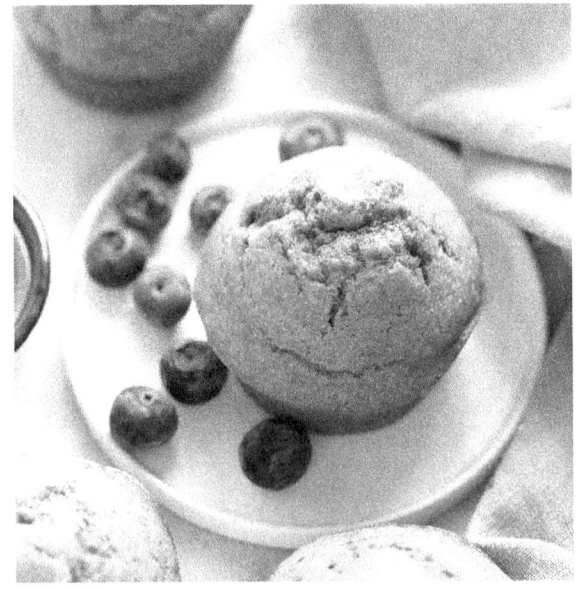

Preparation Time: 10 minutes

Cooking Time: 25 minutes

Servings: 6

Ingredients:

1cups almond flour

1/2 cup powdered erythritol

1 teaspoons baking powder

¼ teaspoon salt

¾ cup almond butter, warmed

¾ cup unsweetened almond milk

2 large eggs

Directions:

Preheat the oven to 350 ° F, and line a paper liner muffin pan.

In a mixing bowl, whisk the almond flour and the erythritol, baking powder, and salt.

Whisk the almond milk, almond butter, and the eggs together in a separate bowl.

Drop the wet ingredients into the dry until just mixed together.

Spoon the batter into the prepared pan and bake for 22 to 25 minutes until clean comes out the knife inserted in the middle.

Cook the muffins in the pan for 5 minutes. Then, switch onto a cooling rack with wire.

Nutrition:

Calories: 135

Fat: 11g

Protein: 6g

Carbohydrates: 4g

Fiber: 2g

Classic Western Omelet

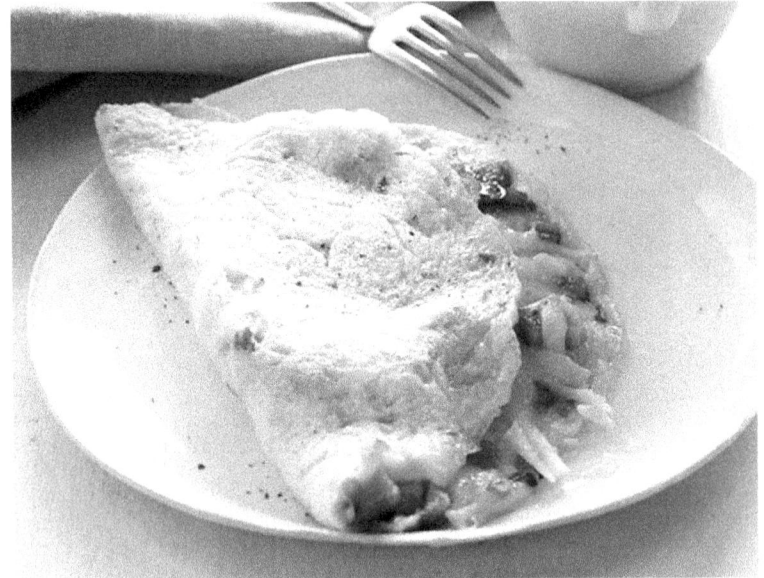

Preparation Time: 5 minutes

Cooking Time: 10 minutes

Servings: 1

Ingredients:

2 teaspoons coconut oil

3 large eggs, whisked

1 tablespoon heavy cream

Salt and pepper

¼ cup diced green pepper

¼ cup diced yellow onion

¼ cup diced ham

Directions:

In a small bowl, whisk the eggs, heavy cream, salt, and pepper.

Heat up 1 teaspoon of coconut oil over medium heat in a small skillet.

Add the peppers and onions, then sauté the ham for 3 to 4 minutes.

Spoon the mixture in a cup, and heat the skillet with the remaining oil.

Pour in the whisked eggs and cook until the egg's bottom begins to set.

Tilt the pan and cook until almost set to spread the egg.

Spoon the ham and veggie mixture over half of the omelet and turn over.

Let cook the omelet until the eggs are set and then serve hot.

Nutrition:

Calories: 415

Fat: 32.5g

Protein: 25g

Carbs: 6.5g

Sugar: 1.5g

Sheet Pan Eggs With Ham And Pepper Jack

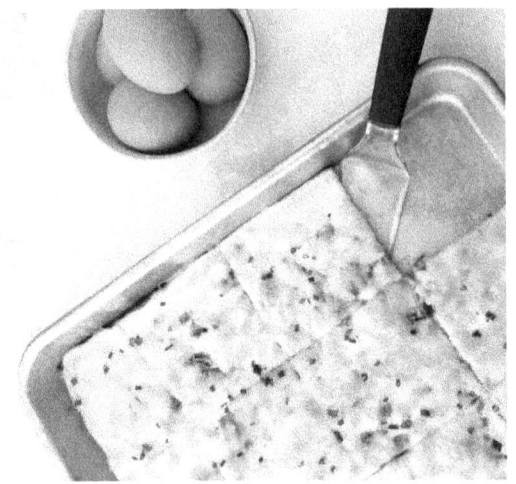

Preparation Time: 5 minutes

Cooking Time: 15 minutes

Servings: 6

Ingredients:

12 large eggs, whisked - Salt and pepper - 2 cups diced ham - 1 cup shredded pepper jack cheese

Directions:

Preheat the oven to 350°F and grease a rimmed baking sheet with cooking spray. Whisk the eggs in a mixing bowl then add salt and pepper until frothy. Stir in the ham and cheese and mix until well combined. Pour the mixture in baking sheets and spread into an even layer. Bake for 12 to 15 mins until the egg is set. Let cool slightly then cut it into squares to serve.

Nutrition:

Calories: 235 - Fat: 15g - Protein: 21g - Carbs: 2.5g - Fiber: 0.5g

Detoxifying Green Smoothie

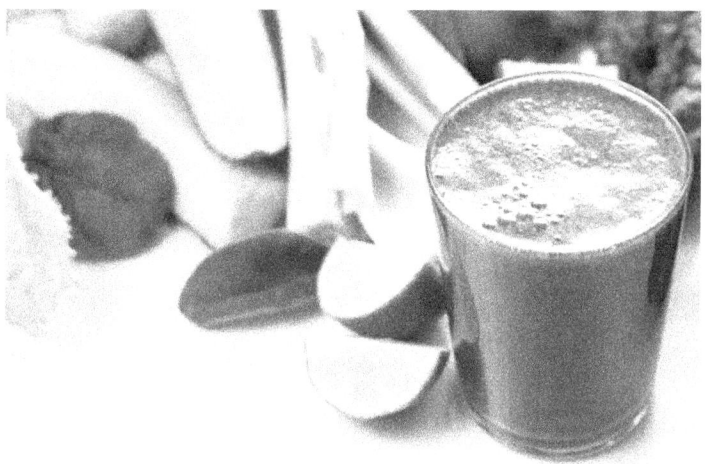

Preparation Time: 5 minutes

Cooking Time: 0 minutes

Servings: 1

Ingredients: 1 cup fresh chopped kale - ½ cup fresh baby spinach - ¼ cup sliced celery

1 cup water - 3 to 4 ice cubes - 2 tablespoons fresh lemon juice - 1 tablespoon fresh lime juice

1 tablespoon coconut oil - Liquid stevia extract, to taste

Directions:

In a blender, add the broccoli, spinach, and celery. Pulse several times over the ingredients. Stir in the remaining ingredients and blend until smooth. Pour into a big glass, and instantly enjoy it.

Nutrition:

Calories: 160 - Fat: 14g - Protein: 2.5g - Carbs: 8g

Nutty Pumpkin Smoothie

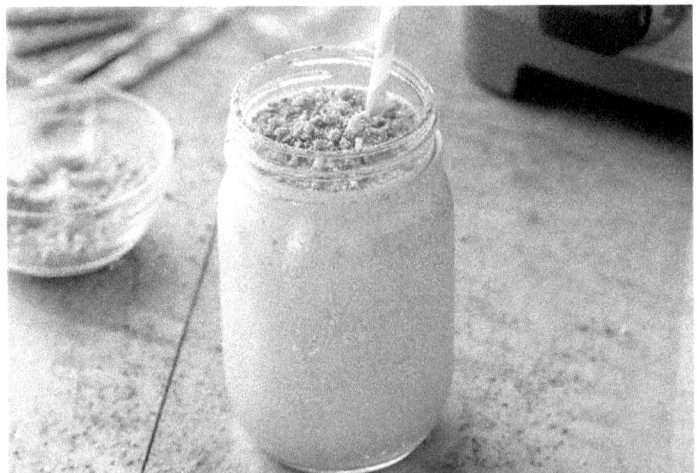

Preparation Time: 5 minutes

Cooking Time: 0 minutes

Servings: 1

Ingredients:

1 cup unsweetened cashew milk - ½ cup pumpkin puree - ¼ cup heavy cream

1 tablespoon raw almonds - ¼ teaspoon pumpkin pie spice - Liquid stevia extract, to taste

Directions:

Combine all of the ingredients in a blender. Pulse the ingredients several times, then blend until smooth. Pour into a large glass and enjoy immediately.

Nutrition:

Calories: 205 - Fat: 16.5g - Protein: 3g - Carbs: 13g - Fiber: 4.5g

Tomato Mozzarella Egg Muffins

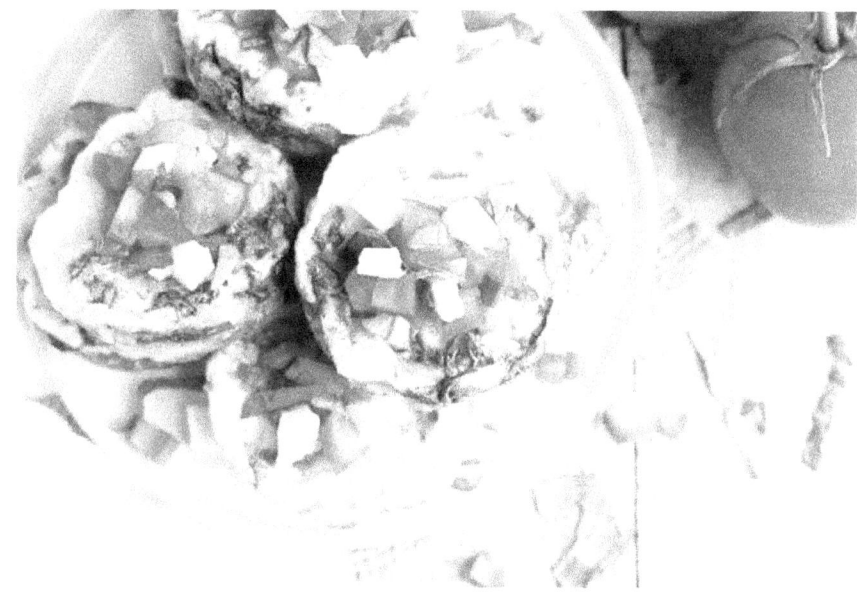

Preparation Time: 5 minutes

Cooking Time: 25 minutes

Servings: 12

Ingredients:

1 tablespoon butter

1 medium tomato, finely diced

½ cup diced yellow onion

12 large eggs, whisked

½ cup canned coconut milk

¼ cup sliced green onion

Salt and pepper

1 cup shredded mozzarella cheese

Directions:

Preheat the oven to 350 ° F and grease the cooking spray into a muffin pan.

Melt the butter over moderate heat in a medium skillet.

Add the tomato and onions, then cook until softened for 3 to 4 minutes.

Divide the mix between cups of muffins.

Whisk the bacon, coconut milk, green onions, salt, and pepper together and then spoon into the muffin cups.

Sprinkle with cheese until the egg is set, then bake for 15 to 25 minutes.

Nutrition:

Calories: 135

Fat: 10.5g

Protein: 9g

Carbs: 2g

Fiber: 0.5g

Crispy Chai Waffles

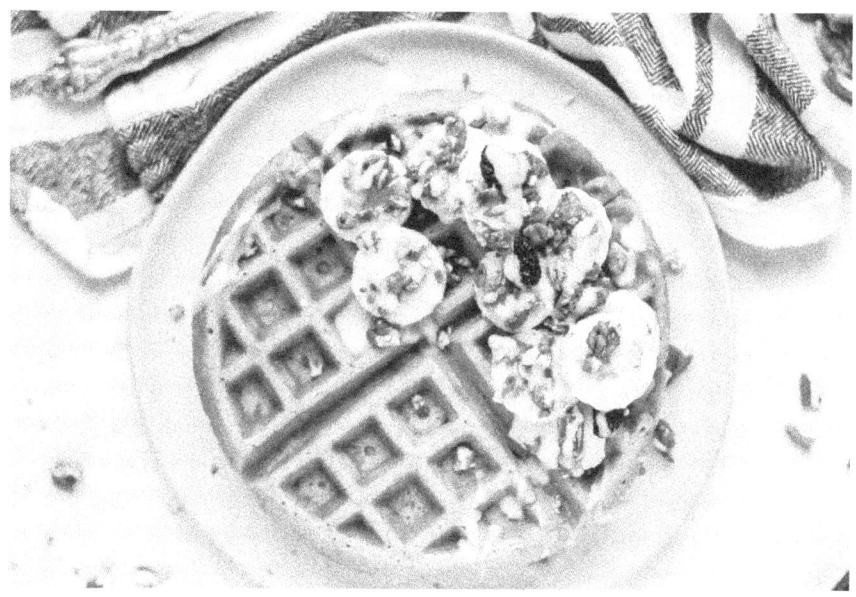

Preparation Time: 10 minutes

Cooking Time: 20 minutes

Servings: 4

Ingredients:

4 large eggs, separated into whites and yolks

3 tablespoons coconut flour

3 tablespoons powdered erythritol

1 ¼ teaspoon baking powder

1 teaspoon vanilla extract

½ teaspoon ground cinnamon

¼ teaspoon ground ginger

Pinch ground cloves

Pinch ground cardamom

3 tablespoons coconut oil, melted

3 tablespoons unsweetened almond milk

Directions:

Divide the eggs into two separate mixing bowls.

Whip the whites of the eggs until stiff peaks develop and then set aside.

Whisk the egg yolks into the other bowl with the coconut flour, erythritol, baking powder, cocoa, cinnamon, cardamom, and cloves.

Pour the melted coconut oil and the almond milk into the second bowl and whisk.

Fold softly in the whites of the egg until you have just combined.

Preheat waffle iron with cooking spray and grease.

Spoon into the iron for about 1/2 cup of batter.

Cook the waffle according to directions from the maker.

Move the waffle to a plate and repeat with the batter left over.

Nutrition:

Calories: 215 - Fat: 17g - Protein: 8g - Carbohydrates: 8g - Fiber: 4g

71 | P a g .

Creamy Chocolate Protein Smoothie

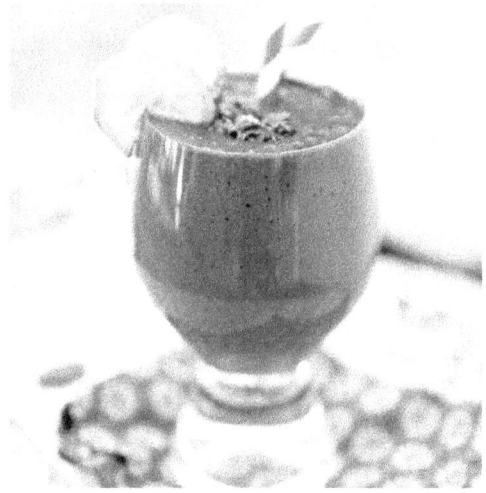

Preparation Time: 5 minutes

Cooking Time: 0 minutes

Servings: 1

Ingredients: 1 cup unsweetened almond milk - ½ cup full-fat yogurt, plain

¼ cup chocolate egg white protein powder - 1 tablespoon coconut oil

1 tablespoon unsweetened cocoa powder - Liquid stevia extract, to taste

Directions:

In a blender, add the almond milk, yoghurt, and protein powder. Pulse several times on the ingredients then add the rest and blend until smooth. Pour into a big glass, and instantly enjoy it.

Nutrition:

Calories: 345 - Fat: 22g - Protein: 29g - Carbohydrates: 12g - Fiber: 3g

CHAPTER 13:

Lunch Recipes

Cole Slaw Keto Wrap

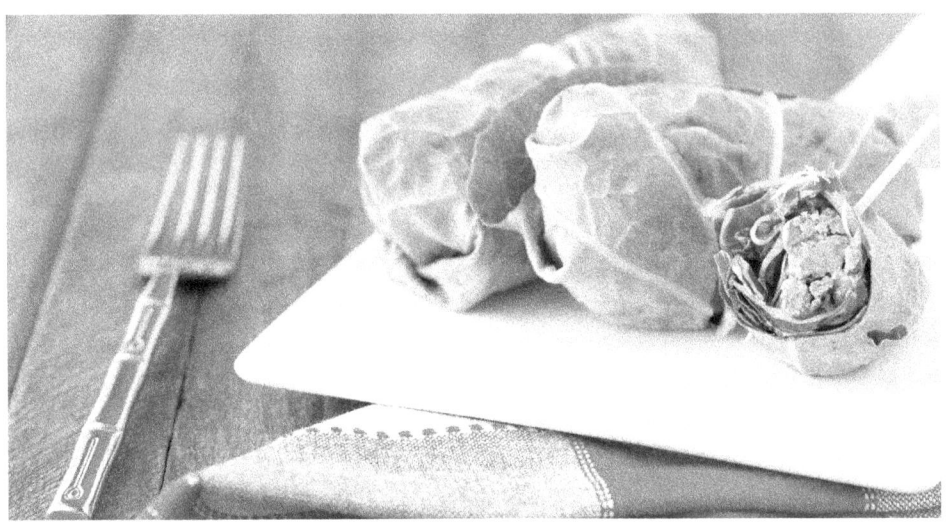

Preparation Time: 15 minutes

Cooking Time: 0 minutes

Servings: 2

Ingredients:

Red Cabbage (3 cups sliced thin)

Green Onions (0.5 cups, diced)

Mayo (0.75 cups)

Apple Cider Vinegar (2 teaspoons)

Salt (0.25 teaspoon)

Collard Green (16 pieces, stems removed)

Ground Meat of choice (1 pound, cooked & chilled)

Alfalfa Sprouts (0.33 cup)

Toothpicks (to hold wraps together)

Directions:

Mix slaw items with a spoon in a large-sized bowl until everything is well-coated.

Place a collard green on a plate and scoop a tablespoon or two of coleslaw on the edge of the leaf. Top it with a scoop of meat and sprouts.

Roll and tuck the sides to keep the filling from spilling.

Once you assemble the wrap, put in your toothpicks in a way that holds the wrap together until you are ready to beat it. Just repeat this with the leftover leaves.

Nutrition:

Calories: 409

Net carbs: 4g

Fiber: 2g

Fat: 42g - Protein: 2g

Keto Chicken Club Lettuce Wrap

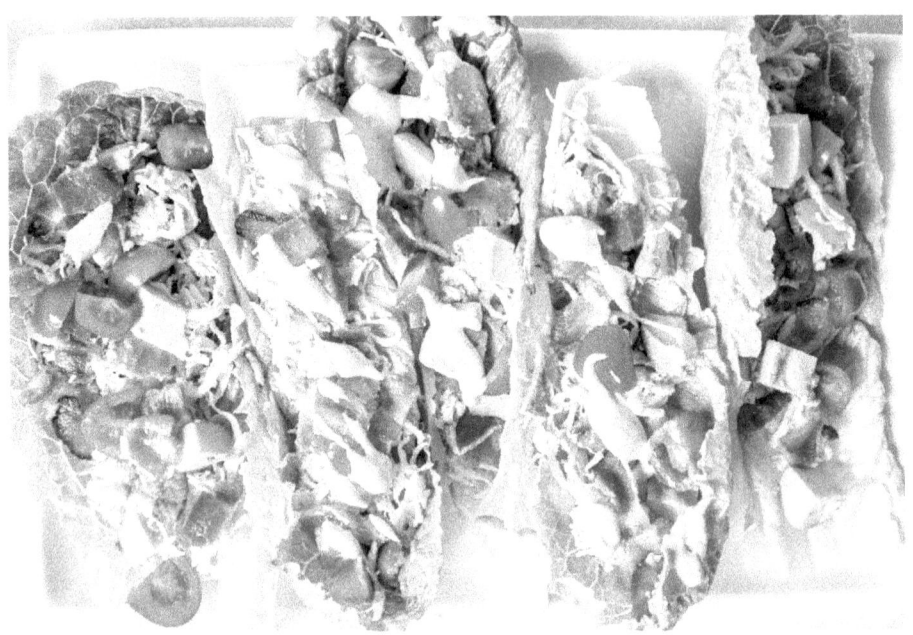

Preparation Time: 15 minutes

Cooking Time: 15 minutes

Servings: 1

Ingredients:

1 head of iceberg lettuce with the core and outer leaves removed

1 tbsp. of mayonnaise

6 slices or organic chicken or turkey breast

Bacon (2 cooked strips, halved)

Tomato (just 2 slices)

Directions:

Line your working surface with a large slice of parchment paper.

Layer 6-8 large leaves of lettuce in the center of the paper to make a base of around 9-10 inches.

Spread the mayo in the center and lay with chicken or turkey, bacon, and tomato.

Starting with the end closest to you, roll the wrap like a jelly roll with the parchment paper as your guide. Keep it tight and halfway through, roll tuck in the ends of the wrap.

When it is completely wrapped, roll the rest of the parchment paper around it, and use a knife to cut it in half.

Nutrition:

Net carbs: 4g

Fiber: 2g

Fat: 78g

Protein: 28g

Calories: 837

Keto Broccoli Salad

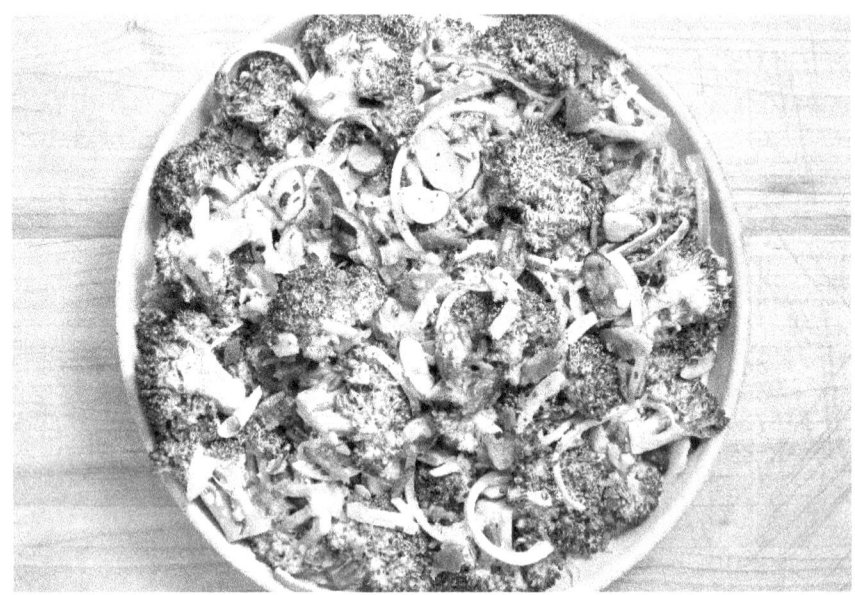

Preparation Time: 10 minutes

Cooking Time: 0 minutes

Servings: 4-6

Ingredients:

For your salad

Broccoli (2 medium-sized heads, florets chunked)

Red Cabbage (2 cups shredded well)

Sliced Almonds (0.5 cups, roasted)

Green Onions (1 stalk, sliced)

Raisins (0.5 cups)

For your orange almond dressing

Orange Juice (0.33 cup)

Almond Butter (0.25 cup)

Coconut Aminos (2 tablespoons)

Shallot (1; small-sized, chopped finely)

Salt (a half-teaspoon)

Directions:

Use a food processor to pulse together salt, shallot, amino, nut butter, and OJ. Make sure it is perfectly smooth.

Use a medium-sized bowl to combine other ingredients. Toss it with dressing and serve.

Nutrition:

Net carbs: 13g

Fiber: 0g

Fat: 94g

Protein: 22g

Calories: 1022

Keto Sheet Pan Chicken And Rainbow Veggies

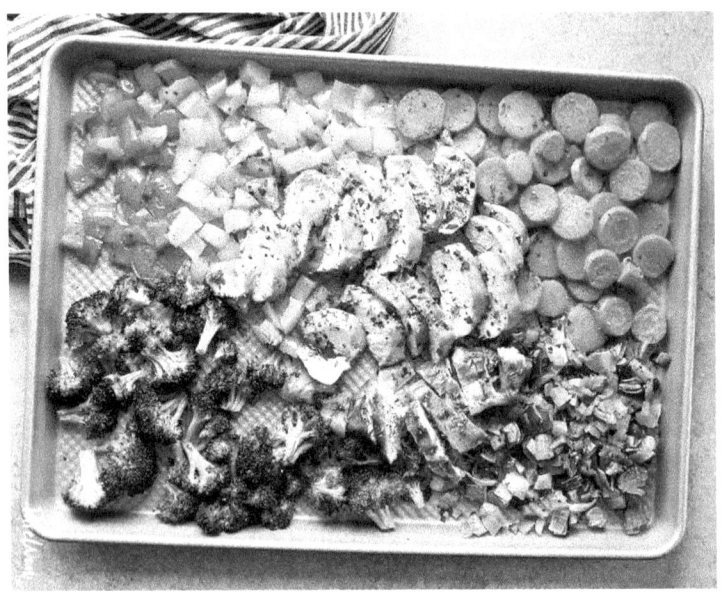

Preparation Time: 15 minutes

Cooking Time: 25 minutes

Servings: 4

Ingredients:

Nonstick spray

Chicken Breasts (1 pound, boneless & skinless)

Sesame Oil (1 tablespoon)

Soy Sauce (2 tablespoons)

Honey (2 tablespoons)

Red Pepper (2; medium-sized, sliced)

Yellow Pepper (2; medium-sized, sliced)

Carrots (3; medium-sized, sliced)

Broccoli (half-a-head cut up)

2 Red Onions (medium-size and sliced)

EVOO (2 tablespoons)

Pepper & salt (to taste)

Parsley (0.25 cup, fresh herb, chopped)

Directions:

Spray your baking sheet with cooking spray and bring the oven to a temperature of 400-degrees

Put the chicken in the middle of the sheet. Separately, combine the oil and the soy sauce. Brush the mix over the chicken.

Like the image above shows, separate your veggies across the plate. Sprinkle with oil and then toss them gently to ensure they are coated. Finally, spice up with pepper & salt.

Set tray into the oven and cook for around 25 minutes until all is tender and done throughout.

After taking out of the oven, garnish using parsley. Divide everything between those prep containers paired with your favorite greens.

Nutrition:

Net carbs: 9g - Fiber: 0g - Fat: 30g - Protein: 30g - Calories: 437kcal

Skinny Bang Bang Zucchini Noodles

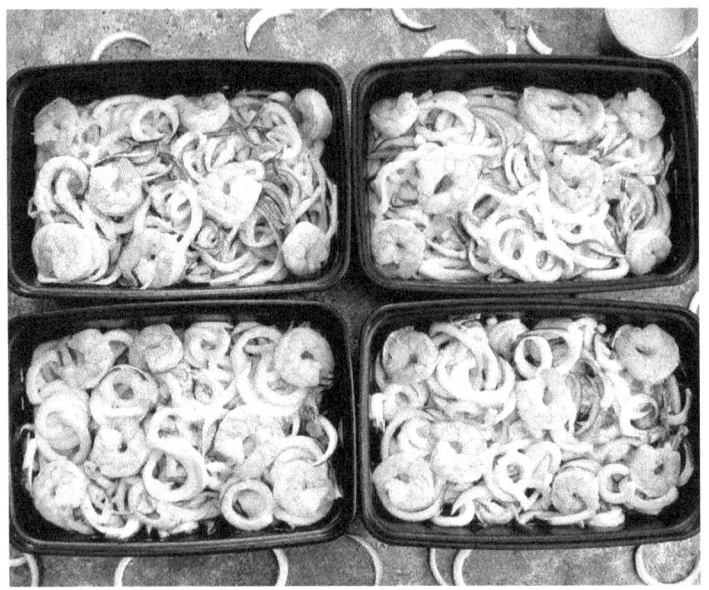

Preparation Time: 15 minutes

Cooking Time: 15 minutes

Servings: 4

Ingredients:

For the noodles

4 medium zucchini spiraled

1 tbsp. olive oil

For the sauce

Plain Greek Yogurt (0.25 cup + 2 tablespoons)

Mayo (0.25 cup + 2 tablespoons)

Thai Sweet Chili Sauce (0.25 cup + 2 tablespoons)

Honey (1.5 teaspoons)

Sriracha (1.5 teaspoons)

Lime Juice (2 teaspoons)

Directions:

If you are using any meats for this dish such as chicken or shrimp, cook them first then set aside.

Pour the oil into a large-sized skillet at medium temperature.

After the oil heats through, stir in the spiraled zucchini noodles.

Cook the "noodles" until tender yet still crispy.

Remove from the heat, drain, and set at rest for at least 10 minutes.

Combine sauce items together into a large-sized both until perfectly smooth.

Give it a taste and adjust as needed.

Divide into 4 small containers. Mix your noodles with any meats you cooked and add to meal prep containers.

When you are ready to eat it, heat the noodles, drain any excess water, and mix in sauce.

Nutrition:

Net carbs: 18g - Fiber: 0g - Fat: 1g - Protein: 9g - Calories: 161g

Keto Caesar Salad

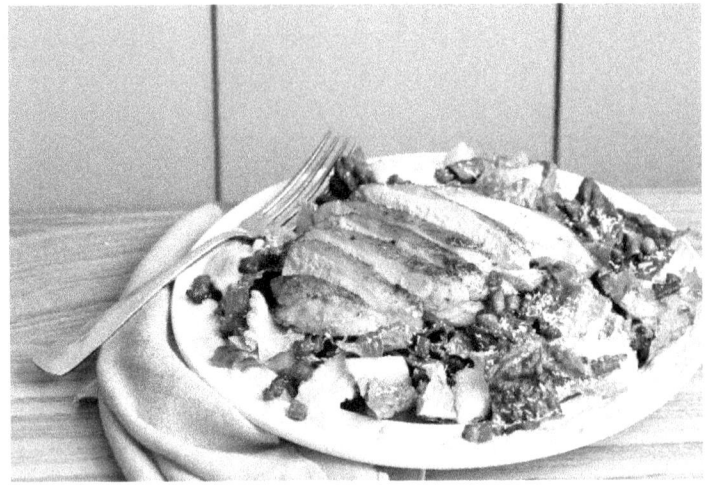

Preparation Time: 15 minutes

Cooking Time: 0 minutes

Servings: 4

Ingredients: Mayonnaise (1.5 cups) - Apple Cider Vinegar / ACV (3 tablespoons)

Dijon Mustard (1 teaspoon) - Anchovy Filets (4) - Romaine Heart Leaves (24 of them)

Pork Rinds (4 ounces, chopped) - Parmesan (for garnish)

Directions: Place the mayo with ACV, mustard, and anchovies into a blender and process until smooth and dressing like. Prepare romaine leaves and pour out dressing across them evenly. Top with pork rinds and enjoy.

Nutrition:

Net carbs: 4g - Fiber: 3g - Fat: 86g - Protein: 47g - Calories: 993kcal -

Keto Buffalo Chicken Empanadas

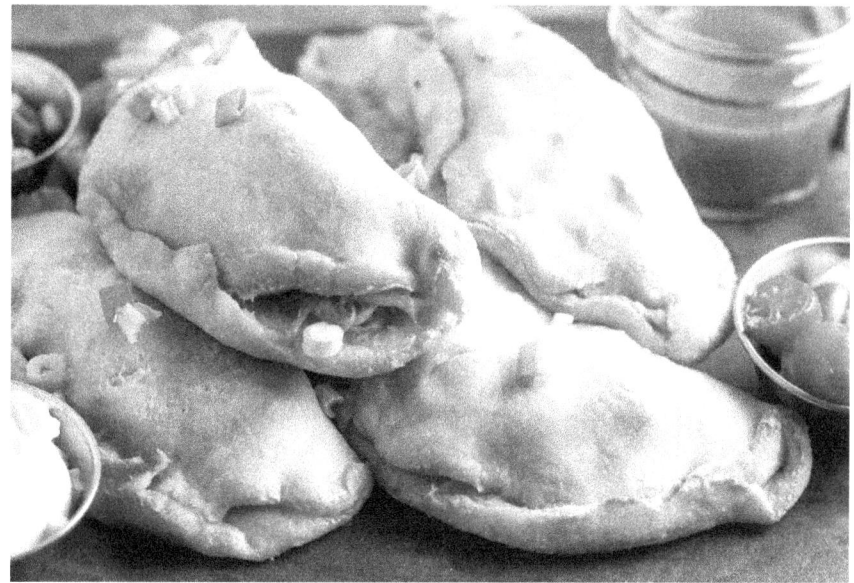

Preparation Time: 20 minutes

Cooking Time: 30 minutes

Servings: 6

Ingredients:

For the empanada dough

1 ½ cups of mozzarella cheese

3 oz of cream cheese

1 whisked egg

2 cups of almond flour

For the buffalo chicken filling

2 cups of cooked shredded chicken

Butter (2 tablespoons, melted)

Hot Sauce (0.33 cup)

Directions:

Bring the oven to a temperature of 425-degrees.

Put the cheese & creamed cheese into a microwave-safe dish. Microwave at 1-minute intervals until completely combined.

Stir the flour and egg into the dish until it is well-combined. Add any additional flour for consistency - until it stops sticking to your fingers.

With another medium-sized bowl, combine the chicken with sauce and set aside.

Cover a flat surface with plastic wrap or parchment paper and sprinkle with almond flour.

Spray a rolling pin to avoid sticking and use it to press the dough flat.

Make circle shapes out of this dough with a lid, a cup, or a cookie cutter. For excess dough, roll back up and repeat the process.

Portion out spoonful of filling into these dough circles but keep them only on one half.

Fold the other half over to close up into half-moon shapes. Press on the edges to seal them.

Lay on a lightly greased cooking sheet and bake for around 9 minutes until perfectly brown. .

Nutrition:

Net carbs: 20g - Fiber: 0g - Fat: 96g - Protein: 74g - Calories: 1217kcal

Pepperoni And Cheddar Stromboli

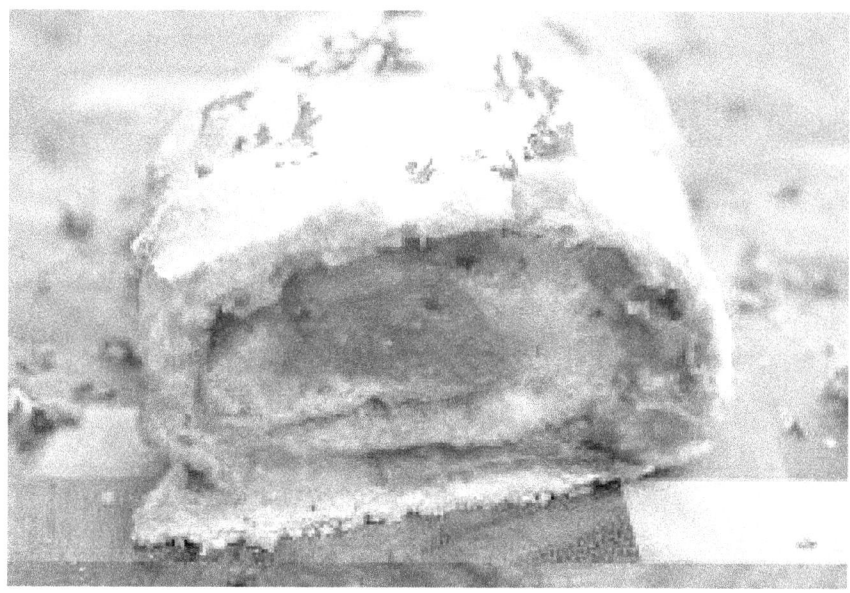

Preparation Time: 15 minutes

Cooking Time: 20 minutes

Servings: 3

Ingredients:

Mozzarella Cheese (1.25 cups)

Almond Flour (0.25 cup)

Coconut Flour (3 tablespoons)

Italian Seasoning (1 teaspoon)

Egg (1 large-sized; whisked)

Deli Ham (6 ounces; sliced)

Pepperoni (2 ounces; sliced)

Cheddar Cheese (4 ounces; sliced)

Butter (1 tablespoon, melted)

Salad Greens (6 cups)

Directions:

First things first, bring the oven to a temperature of 400 degrees and prepare a baking tray with some parchment paper.

Use the microwave to melt the mozzarella until it can be stirred.

Mix flours & Italian seasoning in a separate small-sized bowl.

Dump in the melty cheese and stir together with pepper and salt to taste.

Stir in the egg and process the dough with your hands. Pour it onto that prepared baking tray.

Roll out the dough with your hands or a pin. Cut slits that mark out 4 equal rectangles.

Put the ham and cheese onto the dough, then brush with butter and close up, putting the seal end down.

Bake for around 17 minutes until well-browned. Slice up and serve.

Nutrition:

Net carbs: 20g - Fiber: 0g - Fat: 13g

Protein: 11g - Calories: 240kcal

Tuna Casserole

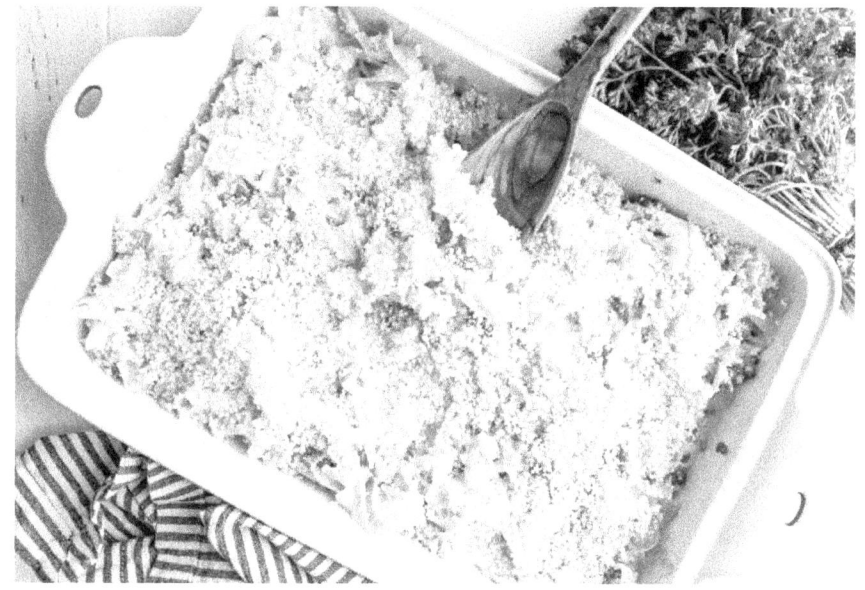

Preparation Time: 15 minutes

Cooking Time: 10 minutes

Servings: 4

Ingredients:

Tuna in oil, sixteen ounces, drained

Butter two tablespoons

Salt, one-half teaspoon

Black pepper, one teaspoon

Chili powder, one teaspoon

Celery, six stalks

Green bell pepper, one

Yellow onion, one

Parmesan cheese, grated four ounces

Mayonnaise, one cup

Directions:

Heat the oven to 400.

Chop the onion, bell pepper, and celery very fine and fry in the melted butter for five minutes.

Stir together with the chili powder, parmesan cheese, tuna, and mayonnaise.

Use lard to grease an eight by eight-inch or nine by a nine-inch baking pan.

Add the tuna mixture into the fried vegetables and spoon the mix into the baking pan.

Bake it for twenty minutes.

Nutrition:

Calories 953

5 grams net carbs

83 grams fat

43 grams protein

Brussels Sprout And Hamburger Gratin

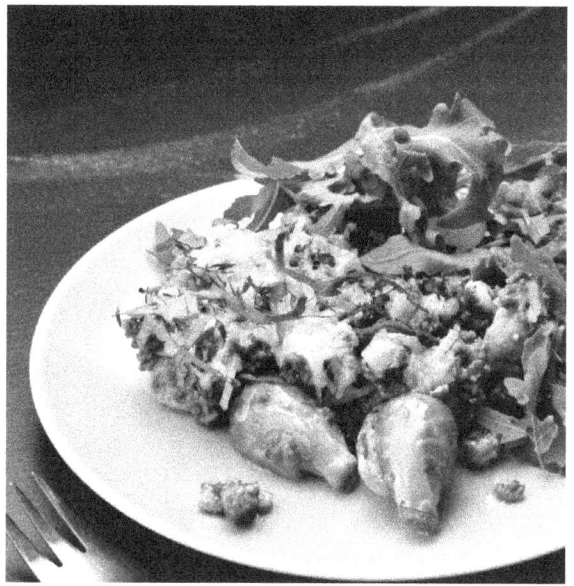

Preparation Time: 15 minutes

Cooking Time: 20 minutes

Servings: 4

Ingredients:

Ground beef, one pound

Bacon, eight ounces, diced small

Brussel sprouts, fifteen ounces, cut in half

Salt, one teaspoon

Black pepper; one teaspoon

Thyme; one-half teaspoon

Cheddar; cheese shredded one cup

Italian seasoning; one tablespoon

Sour cream; four tablespoons

Butter; two tablespoons

Directions:

Heat the oven to 425.

Fry bacon and Brussel sprouts in butter for five minutes.

Stir in the sour cream and pour this mix into a greased eight by eight-inch baking pan.

Cook the ground beef and season with the salt and pepper, then add this mix to the baking pan.

Top with the herbs and the shredded cheese. Bake for twenty minutes.

Nutrition:

Calories: 770kcal

Net carbs: 8g

Fat: 62g

Protein: 42g

CHAPTER 14:

Dinner Recipes

Lemon Butter Fish

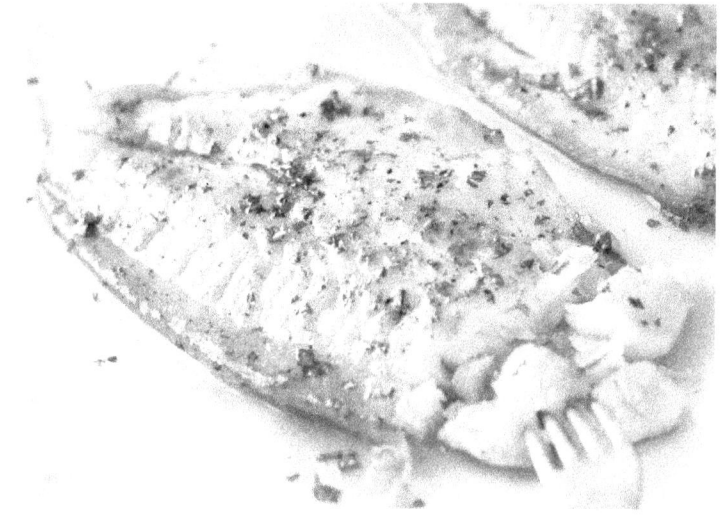

Preparation Time: 10 minutes

Cooking Time: 20 minutes

Servings: 6

Ingredients:

1 tbsp. lemon juice

4 tbsp. butter, unsalted

Sea salt & pepper, to taste

2 tbsp. almond flour

2 tbsp. olive oil

2 tilapia fillets

Sea salt & pepper, to taste

Directions:

Warm the butter in a small pan over medium heat. Warm the butter until it's slightly browned.

Add the lemon juice, pepper, and salt and stir constantly. Adjust seasoning to taste. Set aside while you cook your fillets.

Rinse the fish fillets and pat them dry before sprinkling with salt and pepper.

Spread the flour on a plate or shallow dish and dredge the fillets, spreading the flour over the fillets as needed.

Heat a non-stick skillet over medium heat and warm the oil in it until it's shimmering.

Place the fillets in the pan and cook for about two minutes per side until golden and crisp on either side.

Remove the fish from the heat and place on the plate. Drizzle the sauce over it and serve immediately!

Nutrition:

Calories: 393 - Fat: 28g - Carbohydrates: 3g - Protein: 31g

Chili Lime Cod

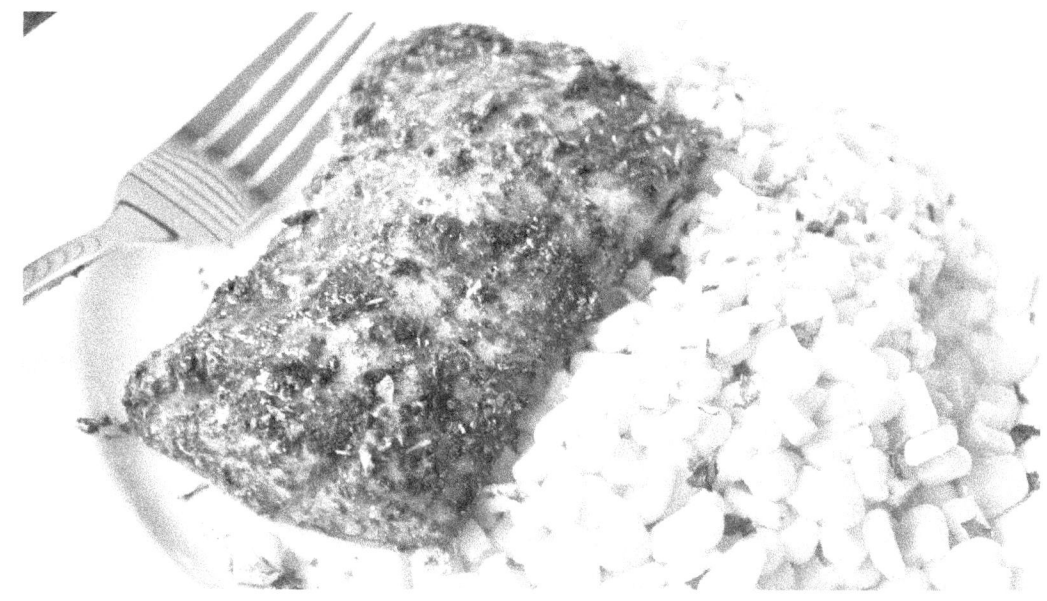

Preparation Time: 10 minutes

Cooking Time: 10 minutes

Servings: 2

Ingredients:

1/3 c. coconut flour

½ tsp. cayenne pepper

1 egg, beaten

1 lime

1 tsp. crushed red pepper flakes

1 tsp. garlic powder

12 oz. cod fillets

Sea salt & pepper, to taste

Directions:

Preheat the oven to 400° Fahrenheit and line a baking sheet with non-stick foil.

Place the flour in a shallow dish (a plate works fine) and drag the fillets of cod through the beaten egg. Dredge the cod in the coconut flour, then lay on the baking sheet.

Sprinkle the tops of the fillets with the seasoning and lime juice.

Bake for 10 to 12 minutes until the fillets are flaky.

Serve immediately!

Nutrition:

Calories: 215

Fat: 5g

Carbohydrates: 3g

Protein: 37g

Lemon Garlic Shrimp Pasta

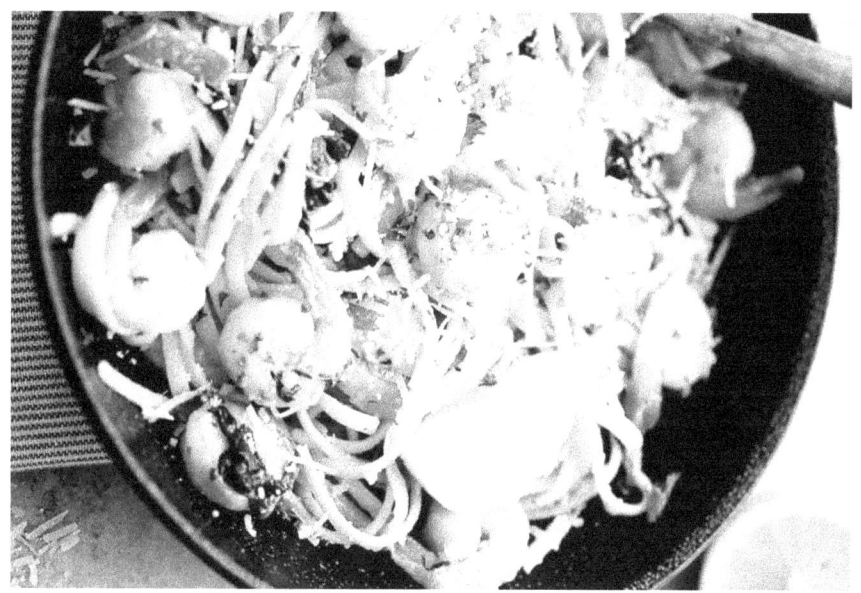

Preparation Time: 10 minutes

Cooking Time: 10 minutes

Servings: 4

Ingredients:

½ lemon, thinly sliced

½ tsp. paprika

1 lb. lg. shrimp, deveined & peeled

1 tsp. basil, fresh & chopped

14 oz. Miracle Noodle Angel Hair pasta

2 cloves garlic, minced

2 tbsp. butter

2 tbsp. extra virgin olive oil

Sea salt & pepper, to taste

Directions:

Drain the packages of Miracle noodles and rinse them under cool running water.

Bring a pot of water to a boil and place the noodles in the boiling water for two minutes before pulling them back out again.

Place the boiled noodles in a hot pan over medium heat and allow the excess moisture to cook off of them. Set aside.

Add the butter and olive oil to the pan, then add the garlic and stir.

Place the shrimp and the lemon slices in the pan and allow to cook until the shrimp is done, about three minutes per side.

Once the shrimp is done, add the salt, pepper, and paprika to the pan, then top with the noodles.

Toss to coat everything together, top with basil, and serve!

Nutrition:

Calories: 360

Fat: 21g

Carbohydrates: 4g

Protein: 36g

One-Pan Tex Mex

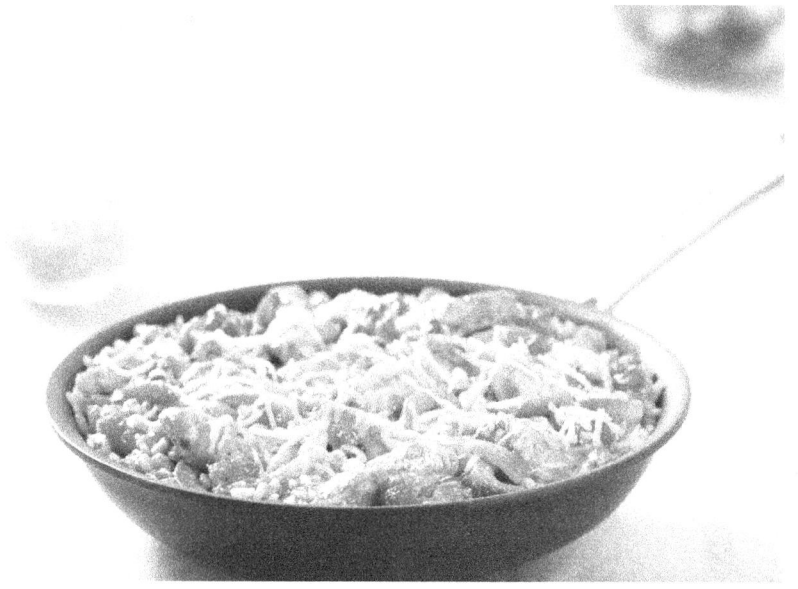

Preparation Time: 5 minutes

Cooking Time: 10 minutes

Servings: 4

Ingredients:

1/3 c. baby corn, canned

1/3 c. cilantro, chopped & separated

½ c. chicken stock

½ c. diced tomatoes & green chiles

½ tsp. garlic powder

½ tsp. oregano

1 tsp. cumin

2 c. cauliflower, riced

2 c. chicken breast, cooked & diced

2 c. Mexican cheese blend, shredded

2 tbsp. extra virgin olive oil

2 tsp. chili powder

Directions:

Slice baby corn into small pieces and set aside. Press any liquid out of the riced cauliflower and set aside.

In a large pan over medium heat, warm your oil and sauté the cauliflower rice for about two minutes.

Add all ingredients except for the cheese and cilantro, and stir well to cook.

Stir in about half of the cilantro and allow the flavors to meld.

Stir about half the cheese into the mix and stir until melted and combined.

Serve and top with remaining cheese and cilantro for garnish!

Nutrition:

Calories: 345 - Fat: 26g - Carbohydrates: 7g - Protein: 38g

Spinach Artichoke-Stuffed Chicken Breasts

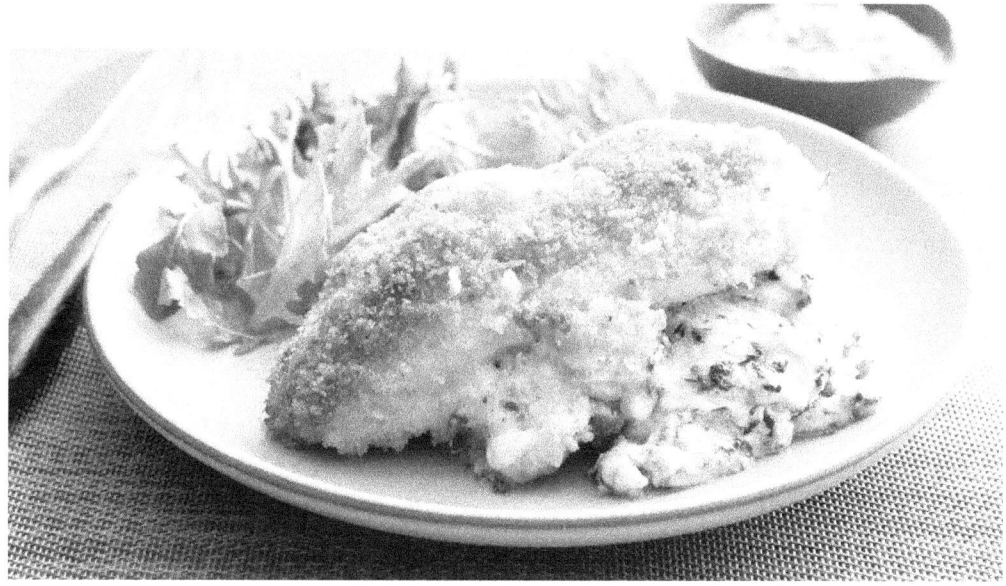

Preparation Time: 15 minutes

Cooking Time: 15 minutes

Servings: 6

Ingredients:

¼ c. Greek yogurt

¼ c. spinach, thawed & drained

½ c. artichoke hearts, thinly sliced

½ c. mozzarella cheese, shredded

1 ½ lbs. chicken breasts

2 tbsp. olive oil

4 oz. cream cheese

Sea salt & pepper, to taste

Directions:

Pound the chicken breasts to a thickness of about one inch. Using a sharp knife, slice a "pocket" into the side of each. This is where you will put the filling.

Sprinkle the breasts with salt and pepper and set aside.

In a medium bowl, combine cream cheese, yogurt, mozzarella, spinach, artichoke, salt, and pepper and mix completely. A hand mixer may be the easiest way to thoroughly combine all the ingredients.

Spoon the mixture into the pockets of each breast and set aside while you heat a large skillet over medium heat and warm the oil in it. If you have extra filling you can't fit into the breasts, set it aside until just before your chicken is done cooking.

Cook each breast for about eight minutes per side, then pull off the heat when it reaches an internal temperature of about 165° Fahrenheit.

Just before you pull the chicken out of the pan, heat the remaining filling to warm it through and to rid it of any cross-contamination from the chicken. Once hot, top the chicken breasts with it.

Serve!

Nutrition:

Calories: 288 - Fat: 17g

Carbohydrates: 2g - Protein: 28g

Chicken Parmesan

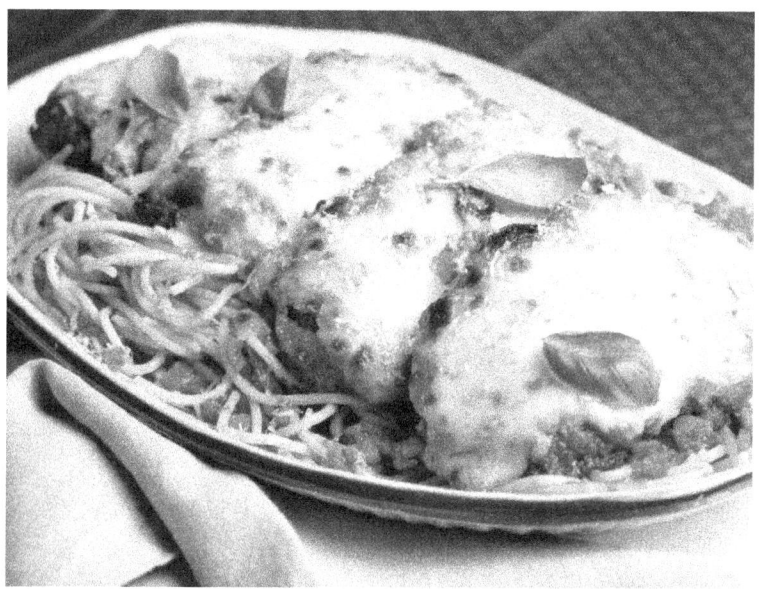

Preparation Time: 20 minutes

Cooking Time: 15 minutes

Servings: 4

Ingredients:

¼ c. avocado oil

¼ c. almond flour

¼ c. parmesan cheese, grated

¾ c. marinara sauce, sugar-free

¾ c. mozzarella cheese, shredded

2 lg. eggs, beaten

2 tsp. Italian seasoning

3 oz. pork rinds, pulverized

4 lg. chicken breasts, boneless & skinless

Sea salt & pepper, to taste

Directions:

Preheat the oven to 450° Fahrenheit and grease a baking dish.

Place the beaten egg into one shallow dish. Place the almond flour in another. In a third dish, combine the pork rinds, parmesan, and Italian seasoning and mix well.

Pat the chicken breasts dry and pound them down to about ½" thick.

Dredge the chicken in the almond flour, then coat in egg, then coat in crumb.

Heat a large sauté pan over medium-high heat and warm oil until shimmering.

Once the oil is hot, lay the breasts into the pan and do not move them until they've had a chance to cook. Cook for about two minutes, then flip as gently as possible (a fish spatula is perfect) then cook for two more. Remove the pan from the heat.

Place the breasts in the greased baking dish and top with marinara sauce and mozzarella cheese.

Bake for about 10 minutes.

Serve!

Nutrition:

Calories: 621 - Fat: 34g - Carbohydrates: 6g - Protein: 67g

Bolognese Sauce

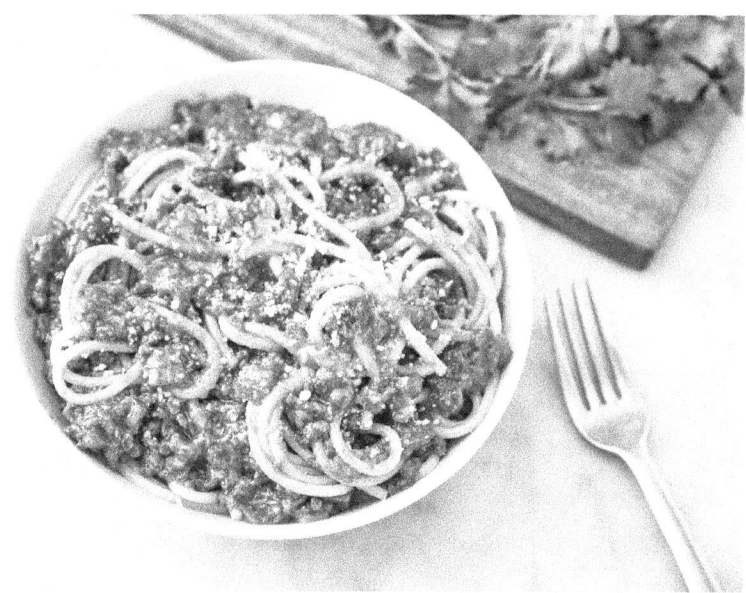

Preparation Time: 15 minutes

Cooking Time: 45 minutes

Servings: 10

Ingredients:

¼ c. dry white wine

¼ c. parsley, chopped

½ c. half & half

1 lg. white onion, diced

1 tbsp. butter, unsalted

2 lb. ground beef

2 med. carrots, diced

2 med. stalks, diced

3 bay leaves

4 oz. pancetta or bacon, chopped

56 oz. crushed tomatoes

Sea salt & pepper, to taste

Directions:

Heat a large pot over medium heat and brown the bacon or pancetta for about eight minutes.

Add the butter into the pot and stir in the celery and carrots. Cook until they're soft.

Add the ground meat to the pot, along with salt and pepper to taste. Break the meat up into chunks as it browns.

Add the wine to the sauce and allow it to reduce for a few minutes.

Add the crushed tomatoes to the pot and stir completely, then add bay leaves, salt, pepper, and stir once more.

Cover and allow to simmer for twenty minutes.

Add the cream to the pot and pull the bay leaves out of the sauce.

Serve!

Nutrition:

Calories: 191 - Fat: 9g - Carbohydrates: 13g - Protein: 12g

Sheet Pan Jalapeño Burgers

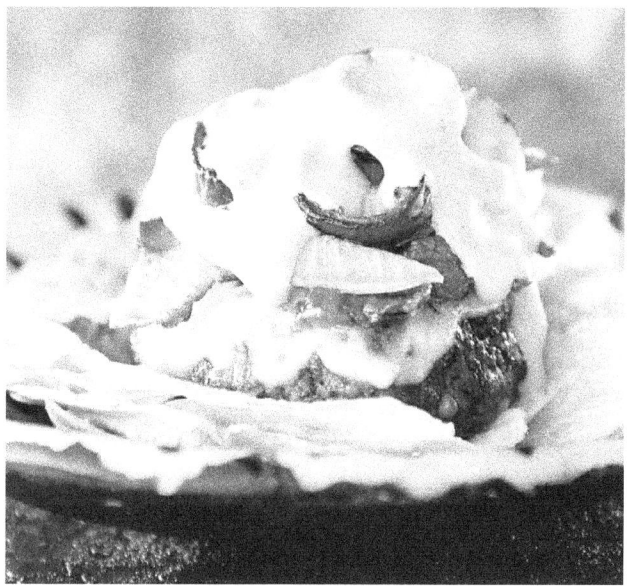

Preparation Time: 10 minutes

Cooking Time: 20 minutes

Servings: 4

Ingredients:

For the Burgers:

24 oz. ground beef

Sea salt & pepper, to taste

½ tsp. garlic powder

6 slices bacon, halved

1 med. onion, sliced into ¼ rounds

2 jalapeños, seeded & sliced

4 slices pepper jack cheese

¼ c. mayonnaise

1 tbsp. chili sauce

½ tsp. Worcestershire sauce

8 lg. leaves of Boston or butter lettuce

8 dill pickle chips

Directions:

Preheat the oven to 425° Fahrenheit and line a baking sheet with non-stick foil.

Mix the salt, pepper, and garlic into the ground beef and form 4 patties out of it.

Line the burgers, bacon slices, jalapeño slices, and onion rounds onto the baking sheet and bake for about 18 minutes.

Top each patty with a piece of cheese and set the oven to boil.

Broil for 2 minutes, then remove the pan from the oven.

Serve one patty with 3 pieces of bacon, jalapeño slices, onion rounds, and desired amount of sauce with 2 pickle chips and 2 pieces of lettuce.

Enjoy!

Nutrition:

Calories: 608 - Fat: 46g - Carbohydrates: 5g - Protein: 42g

Grilled Herb Garlic Chicken

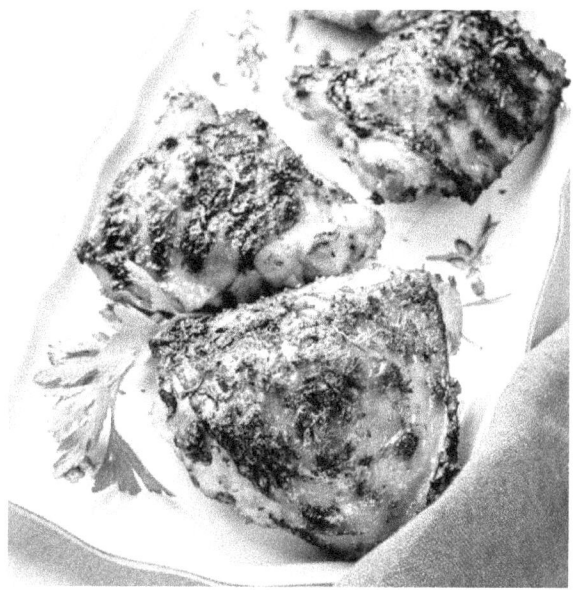

Preparation Time: 5 minutes

Cooking Time: 10 minutes

Servings: 4

Ingredients: 1 ¼ lbs. chicken breasts, boneless & skinless - 1 tbsp. garlic & herb seasoning mix

2 tsp. extra virgin olive oil - Sea salt & pepper, to taste

Directions: Heat a grill pan or your grill. Coat the chicken breasts in a little bit of olive oil and then sprinkle the seasoning mixture onto them, rubbing it in. Cook the chicken for about eight minutes per side and make sure the chicken has reached an internal temperature of 165°. Serve hot with your favorite sides!

Nutrition:

Calories: 187 - Fat: 6g - Carbohydrates: <1g - Protein: 32g

Blackened Salmon With Avocado Salsa

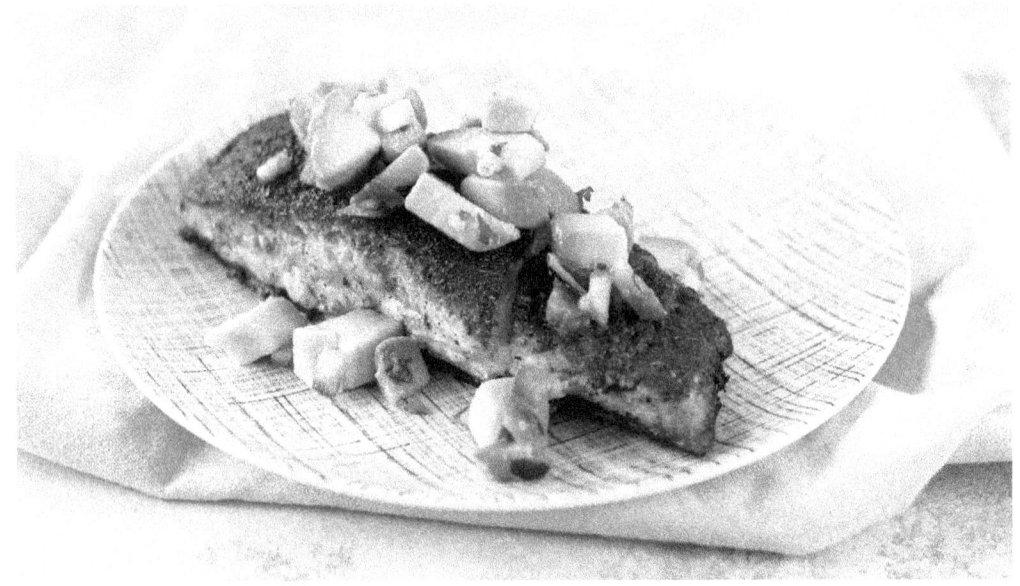

Preparation Time: 5 minutes

Cooking Time: 10 minutes

Servings: 4

Ingredients:

1 tbsp. extra virgin olive oil

4 filets of salmon (about 6 oz. each)

4 tsp. Cajun seasoning

2 med. avocados, diced

1 c. cucumber, diced

¼ c. red onion, diced

1 tbsp. parsley, chopped

1 tbsp. lime juice

Sea salt & pepper, to taste

Directions:

Heat a skillet over medium-high heat and warm the oil in it.

Rub the Cajun seasoning into the fillets, then lay them into the bottom of the skillet once it's hot enough.

Cook until a dark crust forms, then flip and repeat.

In a medium mixing bowl, combine all the ingredients for the salsa and set aside.

Plate the fillets and top with ¼ of the salsa yielded.

Enjoy!

Nutrition:

Calories: 445

Fat: 31g

Carbohydrates: 10g

Protein: 35g

CHAPTER 15:

Dessert And Snack Recipes

Delightful Cauliflower Poppers

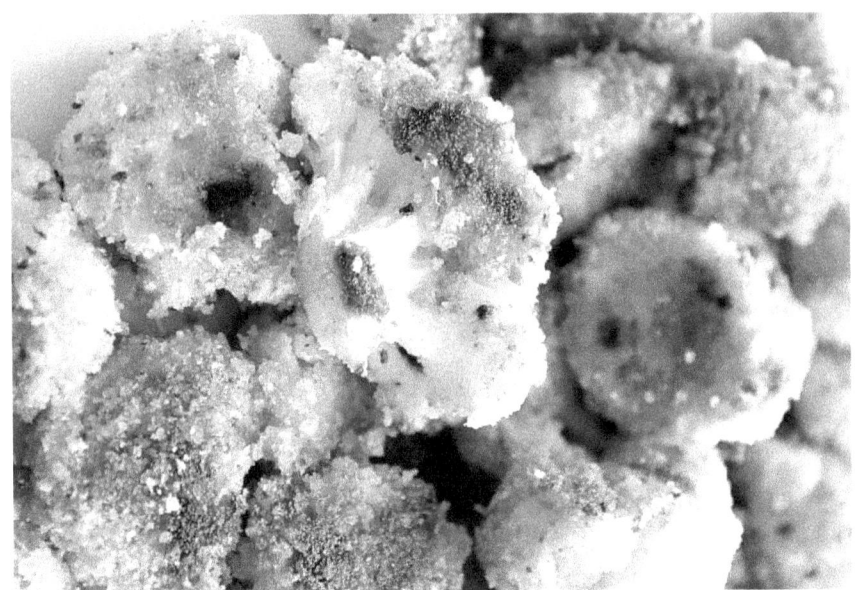

Preparation Time: 15 minutes

Cooking Time: 30 minutes

Servings: 4

Ingredients:

4 C. cauliflower florets

2 tsp. olive oil

¼ tsp. chili powder

Salt and freshly ground black pepper, to taste

Directions:

Preheat the oven to 4500 F. Grease a roasting pan.

In a bowl, add all ingredients and toss to coat well.

Transfer the cauliflower mixture into prepared roasting pan and spread in an even layer.

Roast for about 25-30 minutes.

Serve warm.

Nutrition:

Calories: 46

Carbohydrates: 5.4g

Protein: 2g

Fat: 2.5g

Sugar: 2.4g

Sodium: 32mg

Fiber: 2.6g

Delectable Tomato Slices

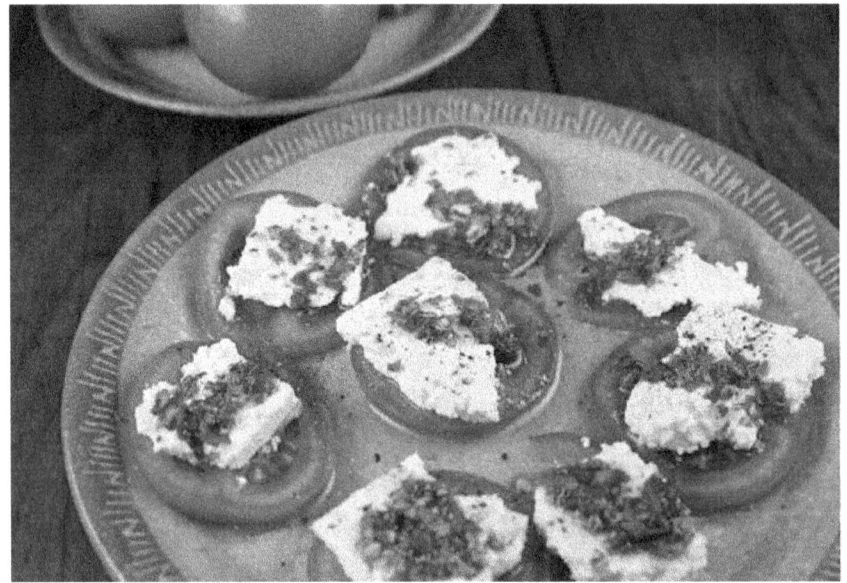

Preparation Time: 15 minutes

Cooking Time: 15 minutes

Servings: 10

Ingredients:

½ C. mayonnaise

½ C. ricotta cheese, shredded

½ C. part-skim mozzarella cheese, shredded

½ C. Parmesan and Romano cheese blend, grated

1 tsp. garlic, minced

1 tbsp. dried oregano, crushed

Salt, to taste

4 large tomatoes, cut each one in 5 slices

Directions:

Preheat the oven to broiler on high. Arrange a rack about 3-inch from the heating element.

In a bowl, add the mayonnaise, cheeses, garlic, oregano and salt and mix until well combined and smooth.

Spread the cheese mixture over each tomato slice evenly.

Arrange the tomato slices onto a broiler pan in a single layer.

Broil for about 3-5 minutes or until top becomes golden brown.

Remove from the oven and transfer the tomato slices onto a platter.

Set aside to cool slightly.

Serve warm.

Nutrition:

Calories: 110

Carbohydrates: 6.7g - Protein: 5g; Fat: 57.4g

Sugar: 2.7g - Sodium: 227mg - Fiber: 1.1g

Grain-Free Tortilla Chips

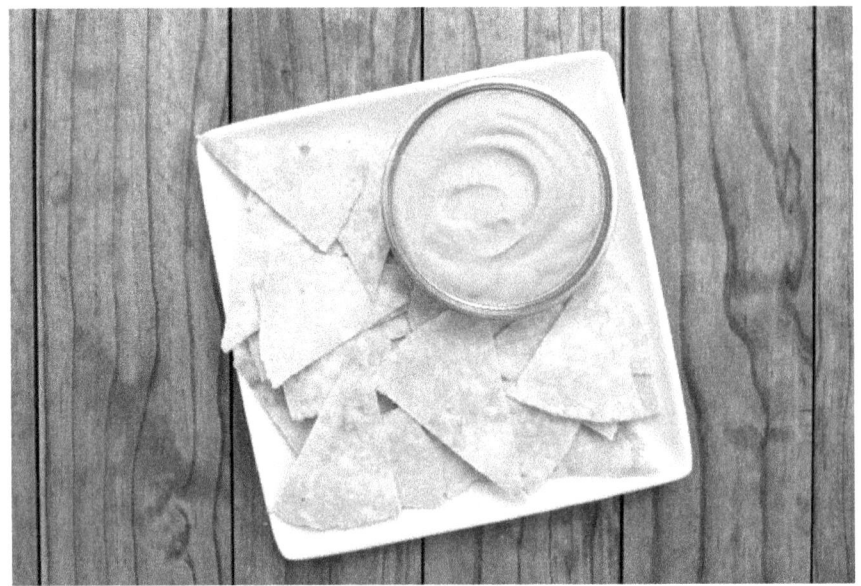

Preparation Time: 15 minutes

Cooking Time: 16 minutes

Servings: 6

Ingredients:

1½ C. mozzarella cheese, shredded

½ C. almond flour

1 tbsp. golden flax seed meal

Salt and freshly ground black pepper, to taste

Directions:

Preheat the oven to 3750 F. Line 2 large baking sheets with parchment paper.

In a microwave-safe bowl, add the cheese and microwave for about 1 minute, stirring after every 15 seconds.

In the bowl of melted cheese, add the almond flour, flaxseed meal, salt and black pepper and with a fork, mix well.

With your hands, knead until a dough forms.

Make 2 equal sized balls from the dough.

Place 1 dough ball onto each prepared baking sheet and roll into 8x10-inch rectangle.

Cut each dough rectangle into triangle-shaped chips.

Arrange the chips in a single layer.

Bake for about 10-15 minutes, flipping once halfway through.

Remove from oven and set aside to cool before serving.

Nutrition:

Calories: 80

Carbohydrates: 2.6g

Protein: 4.2g

Fat: 6.3g

Sugar: 0.4g

Sodium: 70mg

Fiber: 1.3g

Cheeses Chips

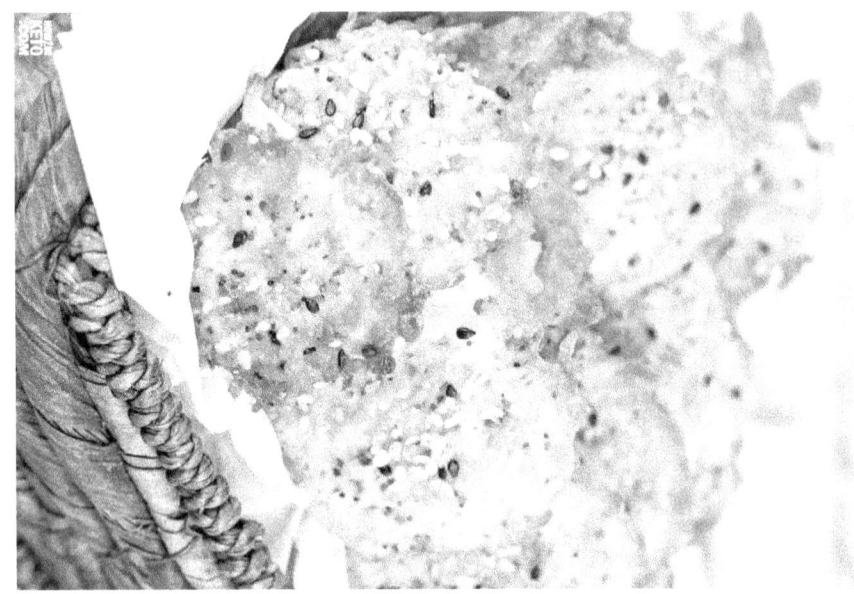

Preparation Time: 15 minutes

Cooking Time: 15 minutes

Servings: 8

Ingredients:

3 tbsp. coconut flour

½ C. strong cheddar cheese, grated and divided

¼ C. Parmesan cheese, grated

2 tbsp. butter, melted

1 organic egg

1 tsp. fresh thyme leaves, minced

Directions:

Preheat the oven to 3500 F. Line a large baking sheet with parchment paper.

In a bowl, place the coconut flour, ¼ C. of grated cheddar, Parmesan, butter, and egg and mix until well combined.

Set the mixture aside for about 3-5 minutes.

Make 8 equal-sized balls from the mixture.

Arrange the balls onto prepared baking sheet in a single layer about 2-inch apart.

With your hands, press each ball into a little flat disc.

Sprinkle each disc with the remaining cheddar, followed by thyme.

Bake for about 13-15 minutes or until the edges become golden brown.

Remove from the oven and let them cool completely before serving.

Nutrition:

Calories: 94

Carbohydrates: 3.2g

Protein: 4.2g

Fat: 7.1g

Sugar: 0.5g -Sodium: 105mg -Fiber: 1.9g

Snack Parties Treat

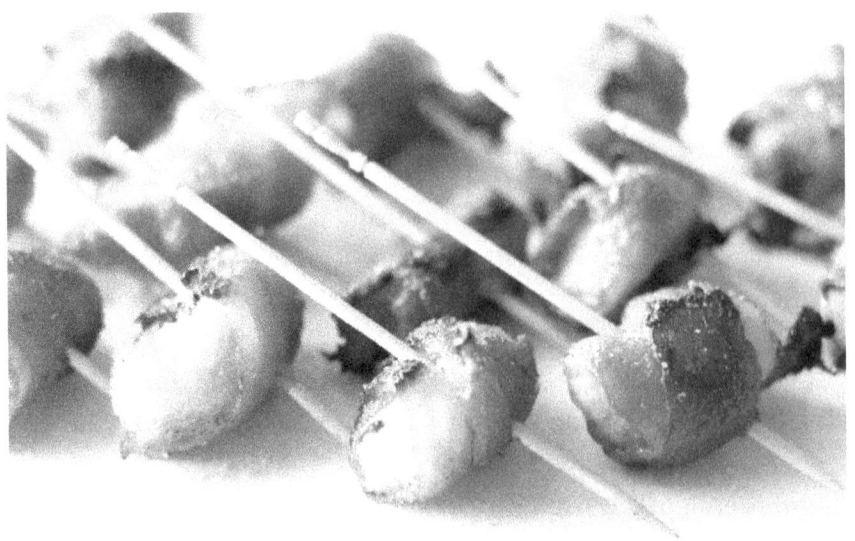

Preparation Time: 10 minutes

Cooking Time: 6 minutes

Servings: 4

Ingredients:

8 bacon slices

8 mozzarella cheese sticks, frozen overnight

1 C. olive oil

Directions:

Wrap a bacon slice around each cheese stick and secure with a toothpick.

In a cast iron skillet, heat the oil over medium heat and fry the mozzarella sticks in 2 batches for about 2-3 minutes or until golden brown from all sides.

With a slotted spoon, transfer the mozzarella sticks onto a paper towel-lined plate to drain.

Set aside to cool slightly.

Serve warm.

Nutrition:

Calories: 906

Carbohydrates: 2.8g

Protein: 37.5g

Fat: 84.6g

Sugar: 0g

Sodium: 1600mg

Fiber: 0g

Sweet Tooth Carving Pana Cotta

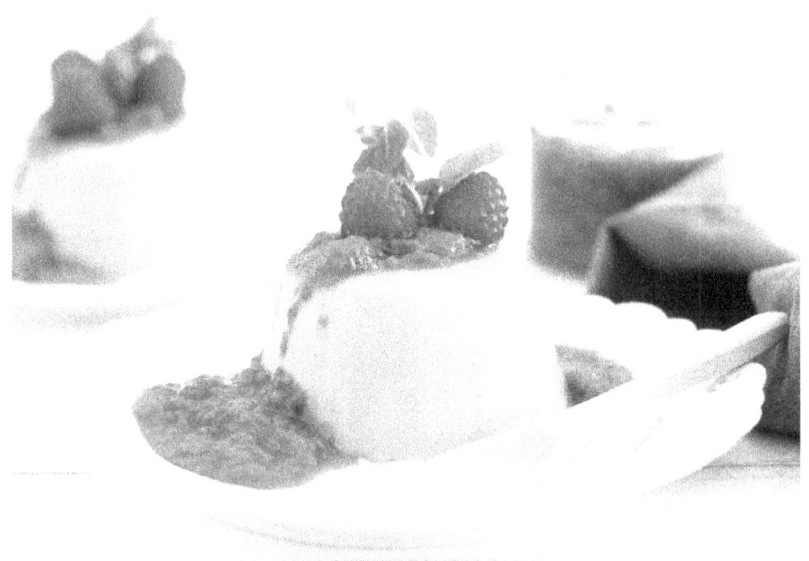

Preparation Time: 15 minutes

Cooking Time: 5 minutes

Servings: 4

Ingredients:

1½ C. unsweetened almond milk, divided

1 tbsp. unflavored powdered gelatin

1 C. unsweetened coconut milk

1/3 C. Swerve

3 tbsp. cacao powder

2 tsp. instant coffee granules

6 drops liquid stevia

Directions:

In a large bowl, add ½ C. of almond milk and sprinkle evenly with gelatin.

Set aside until soaked.

In a pan, add the remaining almond milk, coconut milk, Swerve, cacao powder, coffee granules, and stevia and bring to a gentle boil, stirring continuously.

Remove from the heat.

In a blender, add the gelatin mixture, and hot milk mixture and pulse until smooth.

Transfer the mixture into serving glasses and set aside to cool completely.

With plastic wrap, cover each glass and refrigerate for about 3-4 hours before serving.

Nutrition:

Calories: 136

Carbohydrates: 5.8g

Protein: 4.4g

Fat: 12.1g

Sugar: 1g

Sodium: 96mg

Fiber: 1.5g

Halloween Special Fat Bombs

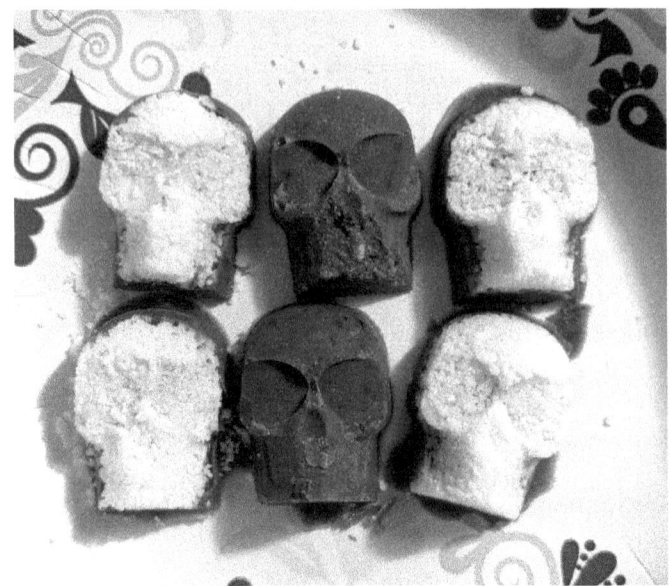

Preparation Time: 15 minutes

Cooking Time: 3 minutes

Servings: 24

Ingredients:

4 oz. cream cheese, softened

½ C. coconut oil

½ C. homemade pumpkin puree

¼ C. monk fruit sweetener

2 tsp. pumpkin pie spice

½ C. pecans, toasted

¼ tsp. ground cinnamon

Directions:

In a medium pan, add the cream cheese and coconut oil over medium-low heat and cook for about 2-3 minutes or until smooth, stirring continuously.

Remove from the heat and transfer the cream cheese mixture into a bowl.

Add the pumpkin puree, monk fruit sweetener and pumpkin pie spice and with an electric mixer, beat until well combined.

Place the mixture into 24 silicon molds evenly.

Top each mold with the pecans, and sprinkle with cinnamon.

Freeze the molds for about 4 hours before serving.

Nutrition:

Calories: 76

Carbohydrates: 1g

Protein: 0.7g

Fat: 8.1g

Sugar: 0.3g

Sodium: 14mg

Fiber: 0.5g

Pretty Blueberry Bites

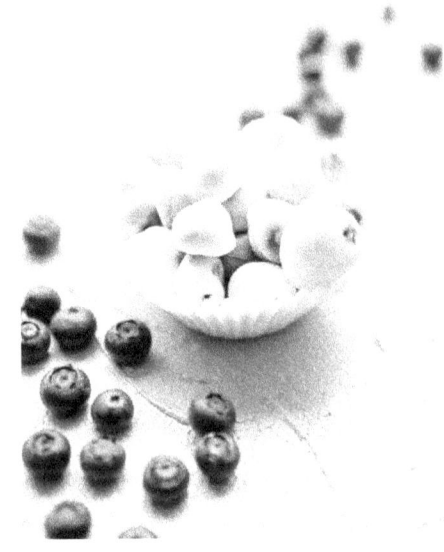

Preparation Time: 20 minutes

Cooking Time: 0 minutes

Servings: 10

Ingredients:

1 scoop unsweetened whey protein powder

½ C. coconut flour, sifted

1-2 tbsp. granulated Erythritol

¼ tsp. ground cinnamon

Pinch of salt

¼ C. dried unsweetened blueberries

½-1 C. unsweetened almond milk

Directions:

Line a large baking sheet with a parchment paper. Set aside.

In a large bowl, add the protein powder, flour, Erythritol, cinnamon and salt and mix well.

Add the blueberries and stir to combine.

Gradually, add the desired amount of the almond milk and mix until a dough is formed.

Immediately, make desired sized balls from the blueberry mixture.

Arrange the balls onto the prepared baking sheet in a single layer.

Refrigerate to set for about 30 minutes before serving.

Nutrition:

Calories: 18

Carbohydrates: 1.3g

Protein: 2.4g

Fat: 0.4g

Sugar: 0.5g

Sodium: 31mg

Fiber: 0.4g

Cold Mini Muffins

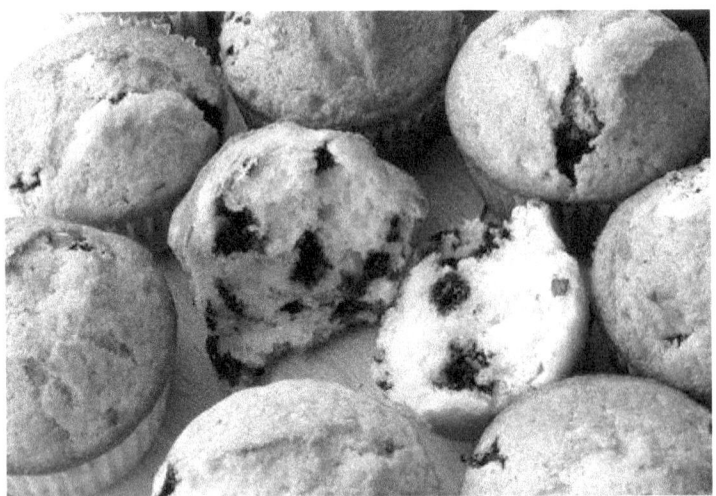

Preparation Time: 20 minutes

Cooking Time: 2 minutes

Servings: 24

Ingredients:

20 oz. 70% dark chocolate chips, divided

¼ C. coconut butter, softened

24 whole almonds

Directions:

Line 24 cups of a mini muffin tin with paper liners. Set aside.

In a microwave-safe bowl, add ¾ of chocolate chips and microwave on High for about 1 minute, stirring once halfway through.

Remove from microwave and stir well.

Divide the melted chocolate into prepared muffin cups evenly and refrigerate until set completely.

In a microwave-safe bowl, add the remaining chocolate chips and microwave on High for about 1 minute, stirring once halfway through.

Remove from microwave and stir well.

Remove from the refrigerator and t top each chocolate cup with the softened coconut butter evenly, followed by the remaining melted chocolate.

Gently, insert 1 almond in each cup and refrigerate until set before serving.

Nutrition:

Calories: 151

Carbohydrates: 7.1g

Protein: 3.6g

Fat: 14.7g

Sugar: 0.2g

Sodium: 9mg

Fiber: 3.7g

Chocolate Lover's Muffins

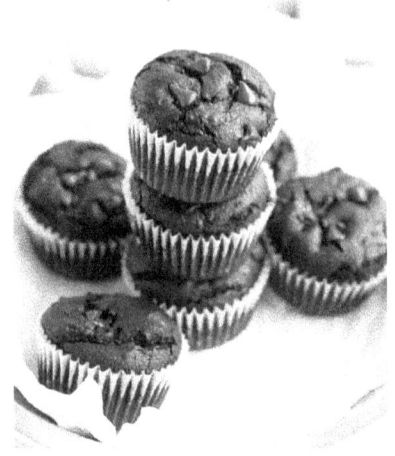

Preparation Time: 15 minutes

Cooking Time: 20 minutes

Servings: 6

Ingredients:

4 tbsp. almond flour

2 tbsp. coconut flour

2 tbsp. beet powder

1 tbsp. organic baking powder

2 organic eggs

1 tsp. liquid stevia

3 tbsp. unsweetened almond milk

½ tsp. organic vanilla extract

1/3 C. 70% dark chocolate

Directions:

Preheat the oven to 3750 F. Grease 6 cups of a muffin tin.

In a bowl, add the flours, beet powder and baking powder and mix well.

In another large bowl, add the eggs, stevia, almond milk and vanilla extract and beat until well combined.

Add the flour mixture and mix until just combined.

Gently, fold in the chocolate chips.

Place the mixture into the prepared muffin cups evenly.

Bake for about 15-20 minutes or until a toothpick inserted in the center comes out clean.

Remove from the oven and place the muffin tin onto a wire rack to cool for about 10 minutes.

Carefully invert the muffins onto the wire rack to cool completely before serving.

Nutrition:

Calories: 151 - Carbohydrates: 10.2g

Protein: 5.2g - Fat: 9.9g

Sugar: 0.7g - Sodium: 223mg - Fiber: 3.9g

CHAPTER 16:

30-DAY MEAL PLAN

Days	Breakfast	Lunh	Dinner	Dessert/ Snack
Day 1	Kale avocado smoothie	Cole slaw keto wrap	Lemon butter fish	Delightful cauliflower poppers
Day 2	Almond butter protein smoothie	Keto chicken club lettuce wrap	Chili lime cod	Delectable tomato slices
Day 3	Almond butter muffins	Keto broccoli salad	Lemon garlic shrimp pasta	Grain-free tortilla chips
Day 4	Classic western omelet	Keto sheet pan chicken and rainbow veggies	One-pan tex mex	Cheeses chips

Day 5	Sheet pan eggs with ham and pepper jack	Skinny bang bang zucchini noodles	Spinach artichoke-stuffed chicken breasts	Snack parties treat
Day 6	Detoxifying green smoothie	Keto caesar salad	Chicken parmesan	Sweet tooth carving pana cotta
Day 7	Nutty pumpkin smoothie	Keto buffalo chicken empanadas	Blackened salmon with avocado salsa	Halloween special fat bombs
Day 8	Tomato mozzarella egg muffins	Pepperoni and cheddar stromboli	Bolognese sauce	Pretty blueberry bites
Day 9	Crispy chai waffles	Tuna casserole	Sheet pan jalapeño burgers	Cold mini muffins
Day 10	Creamy chocolate protein smoothie	Brussels sprout and hamburger gratin	Grilled herb garlic chicken	Chocolate lover's muffins

Day 11	Kale avocado smoothie	Cole slaw keto wrap	Lemon butter fish	Delightful cauliflower poppers
Day 12	Almond butter protein smoothie	Keto chicken club lettuce wrap	Chili lime cod	Delectable tomato slices
Day 13	Almond butter muffins	Keto broccoli salad	Lemon garlic shrimp pasta	Grain-free tortilla chips
Day 14	Classic western omelet	Keto sheet pan chicken and rainbow veggies	One-pan tex mex	Cheeses chips
Day 15	Sheet pan eggs with ham and pepper jack	Skinny bang bang zucchini noodles	Spinach artichoke-stuffed chicken breasts	Snack parties treat
Day 16	Detoxifying green smoothie	Keto caesar salad	Chicken parmesan	Sweet tooth carving pana cotta
Day 17	Nutty pumpkin smoothie	Keto buffalo chicken empanadas	Blackened salmon with avocado salsa	Halloween special fat bombs

Day 18	Tomato mozzarella egg muffins	Pepperoni and cheddar stromboli	Bolognese sauce	Pretty blueberry bites
Day 19	Crispy chai waffles	Tuna casserole	Sheet pan jalapeño burgers	Cold mini muffins
Day 20	Creamy chocolate protein smoothie	Brussels sprout and hamburger gratin	Grilled herb garlic chicken	Chocolate lover's muffins
Day 21	Kale avocado smoothie	Cole slaw keto wrap	Lemon butter fish	Delightful cauliflower poppers
Day 22	Almond butter protein smoothie	Keto chicken club lettuce wrap	Chili lime cod	Delectable tomato slices
Day 23	Almond butter muffins	Keto broccoli salad	Lemon garlic shrimp pasta	Grain-free tortilla chips
Day 24	Classic western omelet	Keto sheet pan chicken and rainbow veggies	One-pan tex mex	Cheeses chips

Day 25	Sheet pan eggs with ham and pepper jack	Skinny bang bang zucchini noodles	Spinach artichoke-stuffed chicken breasts	Snack parties treat
Day 26	Detoxifying green smoothie	Keto caesar salad	Chicken parmesan	Sweet tooth carving pana cotta
Day 27	Nutty pumpkin smoothie	Keto buffalo chicken empanadas	Blackened salmon with avocado salsa	Halloween special fat bombs
Day 28	Tomato mozzarella egg muffins	Pepperoni and cheddar stromboli	Bolognese sauce	Pretty blueberry bites
Day 29	Crispy chai waffles	Tuna casserole	Sheet pan jalapeño burgers	Cold mini muffins
Day 30	Creamy chocolate protein smoothie	Brussels sprout and hamburger gratin	Grilled herb garlic chicken	Chocolate lover's muffins

Conclusion

Thank you for making it to the end. Being on a diet means following guidelines, when you already have guidelines in place, it becomes a process to switch between your current one and your new one. Try not to think about your Keto diet as a lifestyle change that is going to limit you. If you are able to see it as something that is a healthy and positive change, you are going to have a better mindset while beginning the diet. By having a clear understanding of what you should be eating and how you should be feeling, you can compare the way that you feel to the way that the diet is supposed to make you feel. This allows you to stay in control of your diet without feeling that you have to completely surrender all of your decision-making.

We all have our own bad habits, and a lot of us have bad eating habits. In today's society, it becomes easy to fall into these habits because of the promise of convenience. If you had the choice to get takeout or make a meal for yourself in a hurry, you would likely opt for takeout because you have been trained to believe that it is faster and easier. While it might be faster, you are likely compromising the quality of the food that you are eating because it appears more convenient. Most of the time, it doesn't take that much additional effort to cook for yourself. With the way that society pushes fast food and various food delivery services, it is no wonder that you would be more comfortable with allowing someone else to make your food.

While some of these services can be incredibly convenient, you are settling yourself short because you do not know exactly what you are eating. You do not know where the ingredients are from and how they were prepared. These things matter to your overall health, especially as aging becomes a factor. More than ever, you need to be paying attention to the source of your food. When you let these decisions go out of your control, you are allowing others to decide what is best for your body. Even when you begin to feel sluggish and less functional, the body becomes easily addicted to junk food so it will trick you into thinking that you need to keep eating this way.

As long as you have the motivation and the drive to keep moving forward, then you should be able to see real results. It often takes years to form a bad habit, so don't be discouraged if you don't notice a difference immediately. This part does take some time, but each time that you put effort into it, you are going to be working toward your main goal of becoming healthier. Tell yourself that you are doing this for your own benefit. Any time that things feel too difficult, try to get yourself back on track by remembering how great you feel when you are eating natural food that optimizes your health.

The saying remains true — you will realize that what you put into your body is going to dictate how you feel. While on the Keto diet, you are building up energy stores for your body to utilize. This means that you should be feeling a necessary boost in your energy levels and the ability to get through each moment of each day without struggling. You can say goodbye to the sluggish feeling that often accompanies other diet plans. When you are on Keto, you should only be experiencing the benefits of additional energy and unlimited potential. Your diet isn't going to always feel like a diet. After some time, you will realize that you actually enjoy eating a Keto menu very much. Because your body is going to be switching the way it metabolizes, it will also be switching what it craves. Don't be surprised if you end up craving fats and proteins as you progress on the Keto diet — this is what your body will eventually want.

I hope you have learned something!

References

Abrams, R., n.d. Keto Diet.

Baker, T., n.d. Keto For Women Over 50.

Hale, B., n.d. Keto For Women Over 50.

White, A., n.d. Keto Diet For Women Over 50.

CPSIA information can be obtained
at www.ICGtesting.com
Printed in the USA
BVHW061307261020
591816BV00012B/1221

9 781801 125666